Visual Language in Autism

Visual Language in Autism

Howard C. Shane, Ph.D.
Sharon Weiss-Kapp, M.ED.

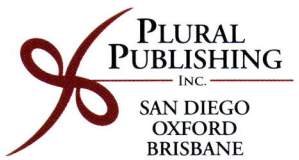

PLURAL
PUBLISHING
INC.

SAN DIEGO
OXFORD
BRISBANE

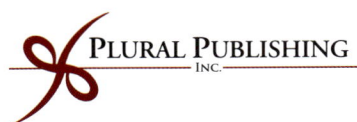

5521 Ruffin Road
San Diego, CA 92123

e-mail: info@pluralpublishing.com
Web site: http://www.pluralpublishing.com

49 Bath Street
Abingdon, Oxfordshire OX14 1EA
United Kingdom

Typeset in 10½/13 Garamond by Flanagan's Publishing Services, Inc.
Printed in Hong Kong by Paramount Printing

Library of Congress Cataloging-in-Publication Data:
Shane, Howard C.
  Visual language in autism / Howard Shane and Sharon Weiss-Kapp.
      p. ; cm.
  Includes bibliographical references and index.
  ISBN-13: 978-1-59756-063-4 (pbk.)
  ISBN-10: 1-59756-063-4 (pbk.)
 1. Autistic children–Rehabilitation. 2. Autistic children–Language. 3. Autistic
children–Education. 4. Audio-visual education. 5. Visual communication. 6. Language
acquisition–Audio-visual aids. 7. Communicative disorders in children–Treatment.
 [DNLM: 1. Autistic Disorder–rehabilitation. 2. Audiovisual Aids. 3. Child. 4.
Communication Disorders–rehabilitation. 5. Language Development. 6. Visual
Perception. WM 203.5 S528v 2007] I. Weiss-Kapp, Sharon. II. Title.
  RJ506.A9S52 2007
  616.85'88206–dc22
                                                                    2007034161

Contents

Foreword

Clinical and basic research related to autism has accelerated at a rapid rate, most dramatically over the past 10 years. First described by Leo Kanner in 1943, autism was initially believed to be related to psychogenic causes. However, by the late 1970s, evidence for an abnormal underlying neurobiology related to the disorder was beginning to emerge. It is now recognized that autism is a behaviorally defined disorder associated with a core cluster of symptoms including impaired social interaction, delayed and disordered language/communication, and isolated areas of interest. Additional features may include repetitive and stereotypic behavior, poor eye contact, disordered sensory modulation, and atypical cognitive abilities. Although there are symptomatic commonalities among those affected with autism, it is now recognized that the disorder involves a spectrum of severity, is clinically and possibly biologically heterogeneous, and may have multiple causes. As a result, what was once known simply as "autism" has come to be referred to as the Autism Spectrum Disorders (ASD).

In 1977, Folstein and Rutter published the results of their twin study in which they noted a substantially higher concordance rate among monozygotic twins than among dizygotic twins, launching the still ongoing search for genetic causes for autism. Although no specific chromosomes have yet been isolated, a number of candidate genes have been identified. Recent studies suggest that the prevalence rate for autism is now 1:150. Although the etiology of autism is believed to be largely genetic, the striking increase in numbers in recent years suggests that environmental factors may also be playing a role.

Imaging and postmortem studies have noted abnormalities in multiple cortical, subcortical and cerebellar regions in the autistic brain. Consistent microscopic findings have been noted in selected regions of the limbic system, regions responsible for learning, memory, emotion, and behavior. Histoanatomic observations in the cerebellum have included significantly reduced numbers of Purkinje cells in many but not all cases. Abnormal minicolumns have been reported in selected areas of the cerebral cortex which, if replicated, could be related to atypical information processing. Increased numbers of microglia and astroglia have been observed in the cerebral white matter, the significance of which is uncertain but which may be related to the presence of abnormal brain circuitry.

Functional neuroimaging studies of the brain have been useful in studying neural circuits and their functions. This technology has been utilized in autism to investigate "Theory of Mind" (the ability to infer the mental state of others) and face processing and atypical connections have been found in these circuits relative to those seen in normal controls. These and other similar studies have led to the hypothesis that autism may be associated with "underconnectivity," particularly in distributed networks as opposed to local circuits. These atypicalities could contribute to the inefficient complex information processing in a number of cognitive and behavioral domains as has been observed in autism.

In addition to abnormal neuroanatomic findings in the autistic brain, a number of neurotransmitter systems have been investigated in postmortem brain tissue, including acetylcholine, GABA (gamma amino butyric acid), glutamate, and serotonin. How these and possibly other neurotransmitter systems impact fetal and postnatal neuronal growth, development and connectivity, and ultimately information processing remains an important and active avenue of neurobiologic research.

There is no doubt that, since 1943, we have learned and continue to learn a great deal about the brain and its functions, both normal and abnormal, and about autism itself. However, there is still much that remains unknown. Further, what we have learned and continue to learn at the basic science level has yet to have a substantial impact on the daily lives of those affected with the disorder and their families. We have come to recognize that early identification and intensive interventional strategies provided to very young ASD children can have a positive impact on developmental outcome. However, we have also realized that autism is heterogeneous and affected individuals can exhibit a variety of strengths, weaknesses, and learning styles and that this is not a "one-size-fits-all" disorder. Thus, although we can now apply general guidelines for treatment and interventional strategies, these guidelines require constant reassessment over time, both in terms of the child being treated and in terms of the field as a whole.

One of the major areas of deficit among those with ASD is language. A child who cannot speak or even communicate nonverbally is a source of frustration for families and for the child himself on many levels. Numerous approaches to communication have been explored and utilized over the years, some more successfully than others. With advances in technology, it has become evident that at least some nonverbal or hypoverbal ASD persons have acquired a good deal of information, may have learned to read and/or solve math problems, and can independently convey thoughts and ideas if given the appropriate communication tools. Some of these tools have been used successfully in classrooms but often have not been utilized in, nor generalized to other environments, making them essentially nonfunctional on a day-to-day basis.

This book offers a comprehensive approach to bridge this gap. Based on their long-standing clinical research relative to communication and success in working with untold numbers of children with ASD, the authors describe a program, known as the Visual Immersion Program (VIP), which combines cognition and language and takes advantage of the child's daily experiences and unusual visual processing of information. The book is well-organized and easy to read, and the methodology is presented in a clear and logical fashion. The authors rightly indicate that "assessment drives instruction" and offer approaches to the evaluation of progress and programmatic changes to meet each child's particular needs. They further provide some specific examples of role-play that can be used to teach the preparation for, transition to, and performance of desired routines. In the final chapter, challenges to working with children with ASD are addressed as well as a brief discussion of augmentative communication devices that are becoming increasingly commonplace within the ASD population.

Given the seriousness and pervasiveness of communication disorders among individuals with autism, and the negative impact that this particular handicap can have on all aspects of their lives, this book offers a timely, comprehensive, multifaceted approach to the development of language and concepts. The book provides creative and concrete strategies for both professionals and parents that should result in a positive impact on the language development of many individuals with ASD.

Margaret L. Bauman, MD
Founder and Director
Learning and Developmental
Disorders Evaluation and
Rehabilitation Services
Massachusetts General Hospital

Preface

When learners with Autism Spectrum Disorder (ASD) first come to our clinic at Children's Hospital Boston, often they are using visual support systems provided by well-meaning educators and families who seem to have only a basic understanding of how visual images can be used to improve communication skills. Over the years, we have seen hundreds of communication books and schedules created by teachers and parents. Although these materials contain visual supports intended to help with expression and organization, they frequently fail to meet this population's complex needs.

In this book, we describe an alternative approach we developed that we believe remedies this problem. Known as the Visual Immersion Program (VIP), our approach provides a comprehensive system of visual representation that links cognition and language in a way that addresses individuals with ASD's unique way of processing visual information and draws from and supports their daily activities in school and at home. As a result, learners significantly improve their comprehension and expression skills, which in turn leads to an enhanced orientation to time and space, better opportunities for social interaction, and more controlled behavior—all of which are challenging areas for learners on the autism spectrum.

The book is divided into seven chapters, each covering critical areas relevant to the VIP. Chapter 1 discusses drawbacks of existing approaches, which typically lie with the underlying conceptual framework. For example, the level of visual representation (e.g., photographs, picture drawings, and line drawings) is often arbitrary, with line drawings the most common choice. Another common problem is that communication books frequently are limited to visuals almost exclusively consisting of nouns and carrier phrases such as "I want _____," which are specifically intended for requesting preferred items. Taken as a whole, these impoverished visual supports create an artificial limit to what students can express.

Chapter 2 reviews fundamentals of communication and language acquisition, as familiarity with these areas is critical when attempting to improve learners with ASD's comprehension and communication skills. Spoken language is a set of abstract symbols that represents conceptual relationships. The VIP provides a systematic progression through visual symbolism, gradually leading the learner from observing basic visual perceptual features to a more profound understanding of language.

Chapter 3 lays out the three primary constructs the VIP: the Visual Expressive Mode (VEM), the Visual Instructional Mode (VIM), and the Visual Organizational Mode (VOM). The VEM uses symbols for expressive communication, perhaps the most frequent application of visual materials. The VIM uses symbols as a sustained referent to support material simultaneously introduced in spoken language, which improves comprehension. The VOM uses symbols to represent the organization of an activity, script, or schedule. We consistently provide research references supporting the efficacy of using visuals in these three modes.

Assessment drives instruction, and, accordingly, plays a key role in this book. In Chapters 4 and 5, we offer a comprehensive assessment that evaluates a learners' performance prior to beginning intervention and offers consistent ways to measure progress. The first assessment chapter focuses on visual skills and other key skills, and the second focuses on experiential knowledge.

Chapter 6 describes our general intervention principles and then details how to implement the three modes of the VIP, using tools such as scene cues, whole scene displays, conversation displays, visual timers, and computer screen displays. We provide a series of lessons and exercises you can use to help learners follow routines, expand language skills,

and increase their understanding of time-related issues.

The final chapter covers a number of important special considerations related to the VIP, including controlling inappropriate behavior, using it in the inclusive classroom and at home, treating learners with severely limited communication and comprehension skills, working with learners with reading skills, and selecting appropriate assistive technology.

Our goal in writing this book is to share our approach with the ever-growing community of people who share a desire to help individuals with ASD maximize personal communication skills, including teachers, teacher's assistants, occupational therapists, speech pathologists, psychologists, and parents. In our experience, professional instructors and parents who use the VIP report that it results in an overall better quality of life for learners with ASD, including improved behavior and increased communication skills. We hope readers also will be prompted to implement the program, leading to similar gains in their schools, homes, and communities.

Acknowledgments

This book would not have been possible without the invaluable contributions of a number of our colleagues. We would like to thank the staff at the Monarch School for Children with Autism in Shaker Heights, Ohio, and particularly Debra Mandell, the school's director, and Jeff Richards, for his contributions in designing materials. Many of the ideas discussed in the book were piloted and fine-tuned in the Monarch School's imaginative educational environment.

We would also like to thank Rebecca Fleisch Cordeiro, for her ongoing contributions to the Experiential Knowledge Profile; Maura Tourian, for her work in what evolved into the Monarch Natural Language Assessment; Jim Sorce for his insight into the application of visual supports; and Meghan O'Brien, who offered her creative talents in designing the graphics throughout the book.

Finally, we would especially like to thank Steven Mardon, for his tireless assistance with the writing and editing. Steve's gift for clarity provided us with the careful and thoughtful framework that made this book possible. He never lost sight of our message and consistently gave us excellent feedback.

Our inspiration for this book and the motivation to complete it came from the children and parents in our clinical practice who live with autism every day. It is our sincere wish that this effort will provide others with a constructive way to improve communication and learning.

To Ron, Ruth, Tim, Marie,
Tony, Mike, Luke, and
Colleen, who continue to
be our inspiration.

1

In Search of a Visually Based Language System for Individuals with ASD

Instructors who work with people diagnosed with Autism Spectrum Disorder (ASD) currently use a range of visually based instructional materials and programs to help them develop and improve learning and communication skills. These methods, most of which emerged in the last two decades, are without doubt beneficial, making it easier for them to ask for items they desire, follow the events in their daily schedule, and accomplish other basic tasks. Successful use of such methods reduces anxiety and frustration, leading to improved behavior (e.g., fewer tantrums, more cooperation, and less acting out).

At the same time, we believe that current methods do not always meet the needs of people with ASD on several levels, thereby creating an artificial limit to what they are able to learn and express. What is needed is an instructional approach that opens the door to much broader communication, enabling them to interact with peers, instructors, and parents in a more profound way. Ideally, such an approach would address three critical areas: (1) language and conversational skills, (2) learning capacity and comprehension, and (3) ability to refer to and orient to time.

Language and Conversation Skills

Ideally, in addition to making simple noun-oriented requests for preferred items (e.g., "I want a DVD"), the individual with ASD would be able to manage

1

Style Notes

For the sake of brevity in this book, we use the term "instructor" to refer to all individuals who work with individuals with autism. Our use of this term encompasses teachers, teacher's assistants, occupational therapists, speech pathologists, psychologists, and, where appropriate, parents. Similarly, we will use the term "learner" to refer to children, adolescents, and adults with autism. Finally, for the sake of grammatical simplicity, we will use male pronouns when referring to individuals with autism, although the principles apply to both males and females.

---

people and events and construct more complex sentences expressing a greater range of thoughts and feelings. He would be better equipped to comment on events and activities around him, respond to questions, and retrieve information from others. Furthermore, he would better understand the relationship between words and concepts, and would gradually develop greater proficiency with expression and comprehension. If possible, he would eventually learn to speak a variety of sentence types, with a range of grammar and syntax and an emphasis on verbs and action-oriented phrases, such as, "I like swimming with my sister" or question, "Why is the dog barking?" In short, he would be able to comment on his surroundings and feelings and relate to other people, closer to the way typical peers do.

Learning Capacity and Comprehension

People with ASD would have less difficulty understanding the content of lessons and would better understand what is expected of them in class. Because these learners often do not understand spoken language or cannot construct meaningful responses to information provided in a classroom setting (whether in a substantially separate or inclusive setting), increasing their learning capacity is often a struggle. Classroom confusion and uncertainty are nearly inevitable. The availability of an approach that clarifies ambiguity about the learner's role and the class material would improve the likelihood of academic success and set the stage for improvements in behavior and social interactions.

Ability to Refer to and Orient to Time

The individual with ASD would be able to understand language in the context of his broader life, so instead of being oriented to the present he would have a greater awareness of past occurrences and future events and make smooth transactions from one setting to another. For example, if a parent said, "We're going to Aunt Sue's house, but first we're going to stop for donuts," he would grasp what this implied for this part of his day. When unexpected developments arose (e.g., favorite teacher out sick, a fire drill, etc.) or something unpleasant lay ahead (e.g., a dentist visit, a long drive), his newfound comprehension skills would enable him to better adapt to the situation. In general, he would have an understanding of what was expected of him at all times; he would have a sense of where he was at any given moment (toward the beginning, middle, or end of an event or task); and he would understand the relationship between his behavior and completing a certain task and receiving a reward (e.g, getting to play a favorite computer game after finishing a learning exercise or a chore).

We have developed a comprehensive visual language approach, called the Visual Immersion Program (VIP), that helps people with ASD achieve these three objectives. As the name suggests, our strategy emphasizes the full complement of possible visual representations —including drawings, text, photographs, television images, video games, computer displays, and objects (timers, toys, etc.), and more. These visual supports are used to link cognition and language in a way that addresses individuals with ASD's unique way of processing visual information, and draws from and supports their daily activities in school and at home. Essentially, the VIP provides the learner with a supplement or alternative to spoken language based on visuals. This visually based system can either serve to bridge the gap to spoken language, or—for the individual who cannot learn to speak—as his or her chief communication method.

The VIP centers on three modes, emphasizing expression, organization, and instruction:

- **Visual Expressive Mode (VEM):** Visual supports used for expressive communication.
- **Visual Instructional Mode (VIM):** Visual supports used an as alternative to or in conjunction with spoken or written language; the intent is to enhance instruction that complements or substitutes for spoken language.
- **Visual Organization Mode (VOM):** Visual supports used to represent the organization of an activity, routine, script, or schedule.

The improved ability to communicate and learn that the VIP provides can have a profound influence on a learner's entire existence: Learning, understanding and expressing, becomes less of a struggle because the individual now has a way to understand and organize his world. Relationships at all levels—between one object and another, between words and concepts, between the present and the past and the future, and between the learner and other people—are strengthened. The learner can better relate to the world of objects and events and find his way to better relationships with family, friends, and the community.

Beginning with Chapter 3, we explain VEM, VIM, and VOM and other fundamental principles of the Visual Immersion Program in detail. In subsequent chapters, we also describe our approach to assessment, which enables clinicians to evaluate learners' communication skills and track their progress; and provide examples of effective visual displays.

It is important to point out that the VIP is not an independent instructional approach or a core curriculum in and of itself. Nor should it be considered a substitute or a replacement for any existing

Existing Programs for People with ASD

Clinicians now use a number of programs to treat people with autism, including the following:

Applied Behavior Analysis (ABA). This approach centers on the theory that behavior rewarded is likely to be repeated. ABA focuses on giving the individuals short simple tasks that are rewarded when successfully completed. Learners usually work for 10 to 40 hours a week one-on-one with a trained instructor, with work usually broken into brief teaching trials. Reinforcers are used to hold the learner's attention, reward appropriate behavior, and promote learning. Each new skill is isolated and introduced alone and then with other concepts.

TEACCH (Treatment and Education of Autistic and Related Communication Handicapped Students). This program is based on the idea that the environment should be adapted to the learner with autism, not the learner to the environment. Teaching strategies rely on intense one-on-one training and visually based schedules and physical structures in the environment to improve communication, social, and coping skills.

Floortime. This approach focuses on a child's play sessions with parents or instructors. Play is a spontaneous, unstructured activity in which the adult follows the child's lead and then elicits and encourages developmental skills. The goal is for the child to learn to connect his ideas and feelings to those of others, leading to emotional growth and increased use of language.

SCERTS (Social Communication, Emotional Regulation, and Transactional Support). This program is based on a highly individualized approach, requiring intervention programs, goals, and objectives tailored to the learner's specific developmental challenges. SCERTS focuses on expanding a learner's capacity to communicate and regulate his or her attention, arousal, and emotional state. Often, professionals from different disciplines collaborate with each other and with families to address a learner's particular needs.

Although each of these programs, and others, can benefit people with ASD, we believe that they can become even more effective when the Visual Immersion Program is integrated into each of these program's particular and unique approach.

educational approach. Rather, it is a supplement to a core curriculum, in which the instructional language we suggest can be used in conjunction with the fundamental teaching objectives. We consider it "agnostic" in the sense that it can be used in conjunction with recognized teaching programs (such as those highlighted on page 4) to help people with ASD dramatically improve their communication skills.

Developments in the Use of Visuals

We recognize that visual supports are already widely used for instruction with people with ASD. Accordingly, it is helpful to examine how visuals currently are used and some of the factors that led to their introduction and adoption. A brief overview of this history can lead to a better understanding of the areas the VIP is intended to address.

In the 1970s and 1980s, researchers made important strides, recognizing key characteristics of ASD and distinguishing it from other developmental disorders. Although some clinical instruction during this time included the use of sign language and some use of graphic symbols (Shane, 1979), efforts to help people with ASD improve communication skills relied almost exclusively on spoken language (and often were only minimally successful).

During this era, relatively few parents of children with ASD sought help from clinicians specializing in augmentative communication. As an anecdotal account, since the early 1980s we have operated a center at Children's Hospital Boston that focuses on severe communication impairment and includes extensive use of speech generating devices and other augmentative communication approaches. Although it is estimated that over half of individuals on the autism spectrum are nonspeaking (Wetherby & Prizant, 2000), in the 1980s less than 5% of our clinical practice included children with ASD. In contrast, such children now make up 50% of our clinical operation.

Facilitated Communication

In the 1990s, several developments sparked an interest in approaches to communication that relied on visual supports. One was the huge amount of attention drawn by Facilitated Communication (FC), a controversial method intended to help individuals with autism communicate. With FC, users point toward a communication device (typically a keyboard display connected to a computer) with assistance from a facilitator who claims to offer only emotional and physical support (Shane, 1994a, 1994b; Shane & Green, 1993).

Although FC has been discredited by the scientific community—a host of controlled studies showed that the facilitator subconsciously cues the user—the attention it drew had the unanticipated effect of helping to legitimize the use of visual supports in working with people who had severe communication problems (including those with ASD). In addition, FC raised parents' expectations of what children with autism might achieve; within a short time span, growing numbers of parents of children with autism started visiting clinics that treated developmentally delayed individuals in search of techniques that would help their children improve their communication skills.

Types of Autism and Prevalence

The fourth edition of the *Diagnostic and Statistical Manual of Mental Disorders* (DSM-IV) identifies five autism spectrum disorders (ASD). The three most common disorders range from a severe form (autistic disorder) to a milder form (Asperger syndrome). If an individual has symptoms of either disorder but does not meet the specific criteria for either, the diagnosis is called pervasive developmental disorder not otherwise specified (PDD-NOS). Two other disorders, both severe—Rett syndrome and childhood disintegrative disorder—are less common.

ASD is four times more likely to occur in boys than girls (CDC, 2007b). All people with ASD demonstrate varying degrees of impairment in verbal and nonverbal communication skills and social interactions, and they exhibit restricted, repetitive, and stereotyped patterns of behavior. In addition, they often have unusual responses to sensory stimuli, events, and objects. The DSMMD can be consulted for full diagnostic criteria.

Recent studies have found higher rates of autism than research from earlier decades, when the best estimate for the prevalence of autism was 4 or 5 per 10,000 children (or 1 in 2000). In 2007 the Centers for Disease Control released data from a 14-state survey that found the rate of ASD was 6.7 children out of 1,000 (or about 1 in 150) (CDC, 2007b). Compared to the prevalence of other childhood conditions, this rate is lower than the rate of mental retardation (9.7 per 1,000 children), but higher than the rates for cerebral palsy (2.8 per 1,000 children), hearing loss (1.1 per 1,000 children), and vision impairment (0.9 per 1,000 children).

There is an ongoing debate about whether the recent data represent a true increase in autism prevalence or reflect changes in diagnostic criteria or increased recognition of the disorder by professionals and parents. Whatever ultimately proves to be the case, it is clear that schools are seeing a sizable increase in the number of children with ASD, and there is a great demand for effective approaches that enhance their ability to communicate. Just as there is a group called Cure Autism Now, or CAN, that supports research on the disorder's possible causes and cures, we believe that parents and professionals should adopt their own motto—TAN—for Treat Autism Now.

Iconicity and Communication Books

Another major development in the 1990s began with researchers making important progress in identifying how people with ASD could best learn new information. A key advance here was the realization that iconic representations were effective as visual supports, and might therefore serve as an effective communication tool. In this context, icons are visual representations, or symbols, that stand for an object by virtue of their resemblance to the object. Research confirmed that the stronger the resemblance between a symbol and what it referred to, the easier it was to learn and remember the symbol (Fuller & Stratton, 1991). Symbols such as photographs and line drawings are usually highly iconic and thus capitalize on the strong visual skills individuals with ASD often have.

The growing interest in visual supports spurred the introduction and rapid adoption of the Picture Exchange Communication System (PECS) (Bondy & Frost, 1994, 1998; Charlop-Christy et al., 2002). This communication approach primarily focuses on a notebook containing symbols depicting nouns. The communicator pulls out the drawings or photos, affixes them to a removable strip on the front cover, and presents an icon or string of icons to a listener. PECS gained immediate and widespread traction with practitioners, especially those oriented toward the applied behavioral analysis (ABA) approach to instruction. Perhaps the greatest appeal of PECS was the approach's simplicity and the ease with which the pragmatic function of requesting could be accomplished through the association between a symbol and a desired object (i.e., manding behavior).

PECS and other notebook-based communication methods that followed represented an important step forward because they gave individuals with ASD an easier way to request their preferences. These methods have several important drawbacks that make them unnecessarily limiting when used as the foundation for a learner's communication.

Restricted Language Function

The ability to effectively ask for desired items and activities is certainly an impor-tant communication skill. Furthermore, being able to successfully make requests often reduces behavioral outbursts and makes a learner more likely to benefit from instruction. However, the constant request for noun-based items, whether in the form of a single graphic or a sentence string such as "I want _____ + _____" sentence structure, tends to reduce all communication to requests, when there is clearly much more to language and social interaction than asking for things. Although parents often place a high value on the number of words in a child's sentence, it is critical to be aware that in terms of communication, saying "I want a cookie, please" is likely no more productive than merely saying "cookie."

Communication books appear to open up a wide range of possible experiences for learners but in reality they are quite limiting. Most of the items fall into a few major categories—foods, toys, tools, body parts, animals, and places. Despite the large number of images, in practice most learners quickly focus on a small number of items and then use them repeatedly. Typically, in our clinical experience, the number ranges from about 10 to 25 items.

Imagine the frustration of trying to express your whole life experience in just a few dozen pictures. For example, a typical display might include pictures of a dozen favorite foods (donuts, pizza, Cheerios, etc.) or a dozen favorite toys (skateboard, video game, Legos, etc), as shown in Figure 1–1. The weakness of such displays is that they do not allow the learner to express more complex thoughts, such as why he likes pizza, or why he doesn't want apple juice today, or how fast he goes on a skateboard and when he last used one. As a result, the

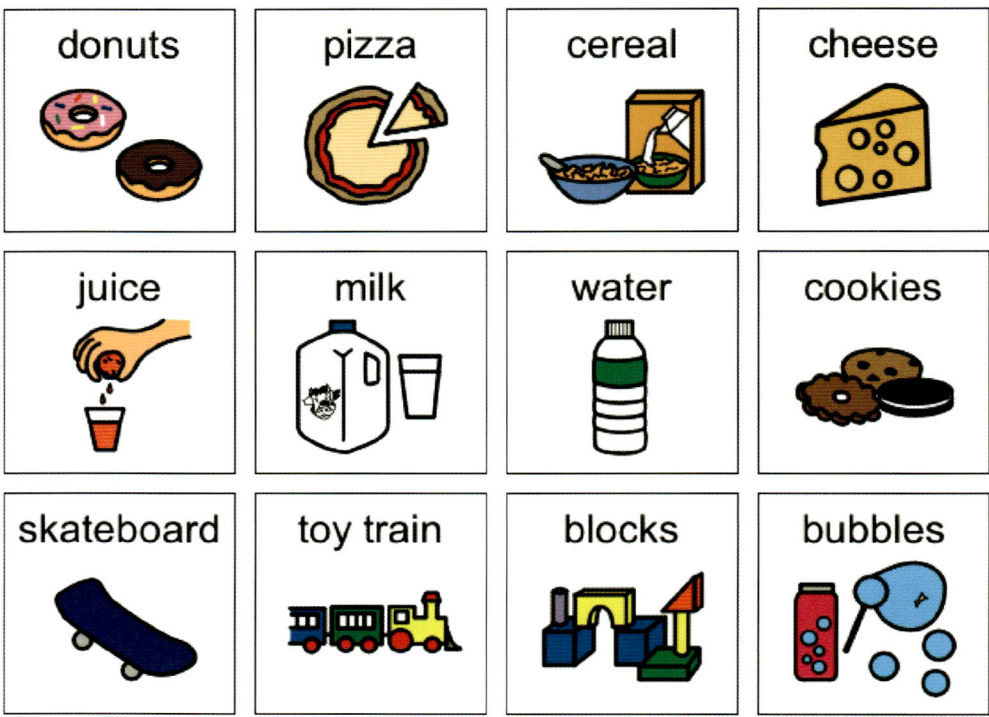

Figure 1–1. Example of typical communication book display (requesting). (From The Picture Communication Symbols ©1981–2007 by Mayer-Johnson LLC. All Rights Reserved Worldwide. Used with permission.)

conversation is liable to end quickly, as there is nowhere else to go once the learner obtains his preferred item. He faces a dilemma: Is there anything else to say once I get my donut?

Restricted Language Growth

Being focused on merely requesting leads the learner to develop an unnecessarily robotic approach to language that is largely focused on nouns (e.g., dog, hand, cup, apple, etc.). He does not learn more complex grammar and syntax that would enable more interactive conversation in which participants expand on each other's statements and transition easily to other topics (such as, "I saw a boy climb a ladder" or "When is grandma coming?").

Focus on Here and Now

Another drawback of "I want _____" sentences is that they are always oriented to the present —what the learner wants at that moment. It's difficult to communicate thoughts and concerns about the past or the future. Many people with ASD have a poor conception of time, which often leads to confusion and frustration. The almost exclusive orientation to the present enables learners only to reference the moment they are in.

Reduced Concept Representation

Another weakness of most communication books is that the symbols (and how they are most commonly used) limit the range of concepts a learner can express. Each symbol is only a rough approximation of the reality of the learner's experience. For example, a picture of a sandwich does not tell him whether his lunch will be hot or cold, what he is actually eating, and what else the meal will include. And a picture of the trampoline symbolizing gym class does not tell him who the teacher is, whether the class is indoors or outdoors, which other children will be there, what today's activity is, and what the teacher expects of the learner. An individual who knows the answers to these questions is apt to be less anxious, behave better, learn more, and enjoy the experience more.

Emphasis on Expressive Communication

Most communication book approaches place their emphasis on expressive communication. Such an approach tends to ignore the importance of comprehension and its role in overall communication growth. Speech, given its ephemeral nature, is not the most effective way to promote information retention. Communication notebooks can offer an effective way of stabilizing a reference to an object in the mind of the learner.

Daily Schedules

The rise in popularity of communication books led to the development of other tools that use visual supports for more specific applications, such as daily schedules (also known as visual schedules and schedule boards). With daily schedules, instructors or parents work with the individual to create a display of words and/or pictures that depict and order his activities for the day (e.g., wake-up, shower, breakfast, brush teeth, bus, school, etc.). Because certain activities change from day to day, the learner may have a series of schedules for different days of the week. Individuals with ASD can help create the displays and also refer to them during the day for information on what is going to happen next, an important tool for reducing anxiety.

Daily schedules represent improvement over the most common use of communication books for requesting items, as they make it easier to address time and tense changes (instead of focusing on the present). However, they have many of the same limitations, such as relatively few items used and limited opportunities for spontaneous conversation exchange, and are thus unlikely to lead to significant language growth and greater understanding of the learner's overall role in his world.

Visual Supports Versus a Comprehensive Visual Language System

All these developments—facilitated communication, communication books, and daily schedules—as well as continued improvements in computer technology, have led to a sea change in how clinicians work with people with autism. It is now clear that visual supports are critical to helping them learn basic communication skills, such as requesting preferred items and following the events of their day.

However, as noted at the beginning of this chapter, although individuals with autism ideally would be able to communicate with peers, instructors, and parents in a more interactive and profound way, often the current use of visual supports does not offer a framework for such progress. The terminology researchers commonly use to describe tools such as communication books and daily schedules is perhaps revealing: They are referred to as visual *supports* because visuals have historically been assigned a supportive role to spoken language. Spoken language is generally viewed as the primary communication system, and visual, gestural, and print systems are typically viewed as secondary support systems. But because some people with ASD often have extreme difficulty with spoken language, a primary system of communication that is based on visuals is needed—one that uses visual symbols not just to support spoken language, but as the foundation for a language system they can use for communication.

The need for an alternative language system becomes clear when we consider how a typically developing child gains language skills. Developmental pragmatics is a theory of language acquisition which suggests that language acquisition is highly dependent on contextual routine-based activities that occur in the presence of spoken language (Tomasello, 1992). Young children begin to interpret the sounds they hear in the context in which they occur, and begin to construct ideas about meaning, structure, and use of the spoken language system.

Typically developing children use language constantly, commenting on the weather, clothes, food, toys, and so forth. They are continuously immersed in language, giving them multiple opportunities to practice, rehearse, elaborate on, and improve language skills. As a result, their ability to communicate their feelings and desires usually progresses steadily.

By contrast, many children with ASD, for reasons we do not yet understand, struggle to process the sounds they hear in a meaningful context. Instead of hearing words and phrases with meaning, they most likely perceive a jumble of disconnected sounds. As a result, they often do not begin to interpret and use the spoken language system, leaving them unable to easily communicate their feelings and desires.

Imagine what it is like to be a child with ASD who cannot speak. Your daily communication is limited to brief opportunities to obtain information or express yourself. Perhaps you have a daily schedule to inform you of your activities for the day. You may also have a display board that tells you how many times you have to perform a task and what type of reward is available for completing the task. If you get frustrated enough, someone may give you a book you can use to point to a finite number of items that you are known to enjoy.

These few instances may represent your only opportunities for communication all day. If you stray from these situational opportunities, your ability to make yourself understood or to understand the intent of others becomes severely compromised. Imagine the frustration of having an imposed limit on your ability to communicate (what we believe is a "communication glass ceiling"). In general, this is what it is like for some people with ASD today.

To compensate for the difficulty that some individuals with ASD have in processing auditory information, they may need a language system in which visuals are used not just to label events or to request specific items, but for sequencing and discussing relationships between events and for commenting on what is occurring. The VIP provides this, helping them to understand the purpose behind a task and the task's specific requirements. They can use visuals to have conversational exchanges that help clarify messages and to tell the story of their day. This provides an opportunity for an enriched language system that is flexible and responsive to the communicative demands of their day.

Compared to current approaches, VIP offers these key advantages:

1. It makes visual symbols—which learners with ASD have an affinity for—the foundation of speech and language acquisition.
2. It uses *all* types of visual symbols, including drawings, photographs, objects, text, and moving images.
3. It makes optimal use of electronic screen displays (on television, computer screen, and video games), providing a dynamic tool for illustrating key language principles, as well as one that learners with ASD enjoy using.
4. Instead of being restricted to output (expression), it emphasizes input (comprehension) as the foundation for communication.
5. Instead of focusing on nouns, it promotes the use of a range of parts of speech and relational

aspects of language (nouns, action verbs, prepositions, adjectives, and adverbs).
6. It allows the learner to easily move back and forth between broad dynamic or static scenes (used for gestalt processing) to single and multielement cues (used for analytical processing).

In Chapter 3, we describe the three modes on which the Visual Immersion Program is based in detail. Before we do so, however, it is important to understand the theoretical basic for our approach. Accordingly, Chapter 2 reviews some key principles of language acquisition and how they are relevant to people with ASD.

References

Bondy, A. S., & Frost, L. A. (1994). The Picture Exchange Communication System. *Focus on Autistic Behavior, 9,* 1–9.

Bondy, A. S., & Frost, L. A. (1998). The Picture Exchange Communication System. *Seminars in Speech and Language, 19,* 373–398.

Centers for Disease Control and Prevention. (2007a). Autism spectrum disorders overview. Available from: http://www.cdc.gov/ncbddd/autism/overview.htm.

Centers for Disease Control and Prevention. (2007b). *Prevalence of the autism spectrum disorders in multiple areas of the United States, 2000 and 2002.* Washington, DC: U.S. Department of Health and Human Services.

Charlop-Christy, M., Carpenter, M., Le, L., LeBlanc, L., & Kellet, K. (2002). Using the Picture Exchange Communication System

(PECS) with children with autism: Assessment of PECS acquisition, speech, social-communicative behavior, and problem behavior. *Journal of Applied Behavioral Analysis, 35*(3), 213–231.

Fuller, D. R., & Stratton, M. M. (1991). Representativeness versus translucency: Different theoretical backgrounds, but are they really concepts? A position paper. *Augmentative and Alternative Communication, 7,* 51–58.

Shane H. C. (1979). Approaching communication training with the severely handicapped. In R. York & C. Edgar (Eds.), *Training the severely handicapped.* (Vol. 4, pp. 155–179). Columbus, OH: Special Press.

Shane H. C. (1994a). Facilitated communication: Why it isn't real. *Clinically Speaking Newsletter, 11,* 1–5.

Shane, H. C. (Ed.). (1994b). *The clinical and sociological phenomenon of facilitated communication.* San Diego, CA: Singular.

Shane H. C., & Green G. (1993, December). Facilitated communication: The claims versus the evidence. *The Harvard Mental Health Letter, 10,* 4–5.

Tomasello, M. (1992). The social bases of language acquisition. *Social Development, 1,* 67–87.

Wetherby, A., & Prizant, B. (2000). *Autism spectrum disorders: A transactional developmental perspective.* Baltimore: Brookes.

2

Fundamentals of Communication and Language Acquisition

We encounter thousands of symbols every day and, without giving it much thought, process them with our ears and eyes. Our ability to derive meaning from symbols enables us to read, speak, listen, and find our way around, which in turn allows us to work, converse with friends, shop, enjoy entertainment, and generally live our lives. This occurs so naturally that we may overlook how complex the process of interpreting symbols really is, as well as the rapid progress we made early in life in learning to make our thoughts and feelings clear. Consider, for example, the obvious differences in communication skills between a new-born baby, a 2-year-old, a 5-year-old, and a 10-year-old.

In this chapter, we briefly review the language fundamentals that enable a child to learn to communicate. As we do so, we highlight how each element relates to individuals with ASD. Such a review, although not intended to be exhaustive, helps lay the foundation for the three modes upon which the Visual Immersion Program is based.

Symbols

Symbols play a critical role in most communication, so we begin by discussing their function and how people use them. A symbol is defined as something that stands for something else and is used with a specific intention. Symbols, which can be verbal and nonverbal, are used to represent words, objects, concepts, events, actions, and so on. These words, objects, and so forth that symbols refer to are called referents.

We live in a symbol-rich environment. Consider, for example, the many symbols you encounter on a trip to the supermarket. Between announcements on the PA system, product logos, product names, and the body language of other customers, you are literally inundated with thousands of symbols. The large number of symbols we encounter on a daily basis can be broken into four types: gestural, visual, spoken, and graphic:

Gestural Symbols

Gestural symbols are body movements used to represent words or actions, such as waving one's hands to symbolize "come over here" or pointing to mean "look at that." Gestural communication relies on a shared understanding of what the gesture symbolizes. When someone shrugs his shoulders, he intends to communicate "I don't know," but the intent is only transmitted if the communication partner shares knowledge of this gesture's meaning. Facial expressions such as smiles or frowns (also known as affect) also are a form of gestural symbols, as are the hand gestures used in

sign language (see Sign Language and Learners with ASD below).

Individuals with ASD are often slow to develop the ability to use and recognize gestural symbols. For example, they may lag at activities involving "joint attention"—when two people look at the same target after one has pointed to it. Joint attention is considered a predictive indicator of language acquisition because it requires that the learner see another person's communication as mindful and intentional (Wetherby et al., 1998). Compared to typically developing children, children with autism are less likely to look at objects or persons that are pointed to. They are also less likely to point in order to capture another's attention (Wetherby et al., 1998).

Learners with ASD also are less able to "read" the faces of other people than their typically developing peers. However, they are able to interpret the social-perceptual aspects of emotion (e.g., posture, facial expression, sound of voice), but have difficulty associating these perceptual characteristics with the more complex cognitive domains associated

---

Sign Language and Learners with ASD

In our clinical practice we often see learners with ASD who have successfully learned a number of signs, and this had a positive affect on their lives. For example, they may be able to use sign language to communicate concepts such as "I'm tired" and "I want a glass of water." Basic competence with sign language can reduce frustration associated with not being able to specify desired items.

Despite sign language's initial effectiveness, we have found that learners with ASD can generally learn to use well-chosen visual symbols more easily than they can learn to use the gestural symbols of sign language. Most likely this is due to visual symbols' high iconicity. In other words, it is easier for a learner to make the connection between a picture of a tree and a real tree than to make the connection between the sign language hand symbol for a tree and a real tree.

with them. They may not, for example, access language and experiential knowledge to connect that Mommy looks upset *because* she can't find her keys and is late for work. Such difficulty recognizing the emotional states of other people can lead to problems in social situations.

Note that gestural symbols are different from physical reenactments—anticipatory linear repetitions of a single event (Wetherby & Prizant, 2000). Examples include a child retrieving an object on his own after seeing an adult obtain it from the same place earlier and a child grabbing his mother's hand and physically leading her to the site. Because the desired object has to be accessible to be retrieved, such re-enactments are nonsymbolic, that is, no symbol is replacing another object or concept. Physical re-enactments are therefore a limited communication mode, as anything that is out of view is unattainable.

Visual Symbols

There are many types of visual symbols, such as drawings, photographs, and text (see Levels of Visual Representation on the following page). Objects also can serve as visual symbols; for example, a doll may be a symbol for a person, and dollhouse furniture may stand for furniture in the natural environment. Visual symbols are effective tools for conveying and clarifying meaning, even at a young age. For example, a 2-year-old quickly grasps that the golden arches logo symbolizes McDonald's, and may become excited at the possibility of having a favorite meal or being part of the overall McDonald's experience when seeing this symbol. Many of us find it helpful when the directions for constructing a desk or a bicycle

come with pictures as visual supports. Photographs, too, are effective symbols, helping us remember events from our own lives and important scenes from history. Photographs can prepare us for the requirements of a novel situation (such as planning a first visit to a town).

As noted in Chapter 1, individuals with ASD often do well interpreting visual symbols because they convey a wide range of information and effectively represent basic words and concepts. As a result, visual symbols are widely used to help learners with ASD make requests and chart the events of their day, and are the chief symbol type used in the VIP.

Spoken Symbols

When we speak, we put sounds together to form words, which are used to represent things and express concepts and ideas. When one person says the word "pen" or "running" or "democracy," someone who shares the same spoken language system knows what this suggests. For communication to occur, however, the speaker's intention and the listener's understanding must substantially match. Note that spoken symbols are not universally consistent. Different languages have different words for the same object, that is, "pen," "le stylo" (French), and "la pluma" (Spanish) all symbolize the same object. For communication to occur, "pen" has to mean an "instrument for writing" to all parties.

Learners with ASD often have difficulty understanding the meaning of spoken symbols or difficulty processing them. Although their hearing is not impaired, they struggle to break down the stream of sounds they are hearing into meaningful words and phrases, limiting

Levels of Visual Representation

There are several ways of classifying visual symbols, but we find it most useful to put them in the following categories:

- A **proxy** is using one physical object to substitute for another object. For example, an empty box of Cheerios can serve as a proxy for a full box.
- **3D photographs** are a tool we use that combines photos and objects. For example, one can cut out the front cover of a cereal box or picture of a toy (with background removed) and paste it onto foam board that is approximately the same size as the actual cereal box. 3D photographs look more like an object than traditional two-dimensional photos.
- **2D photographs** are ordinary two-dimensional photos, such as snapshots or the photographs found in a magazine. (We will refer to these as photos.)
- **Pictures** are detailed drawings that very closely depict an item. Such pictures are usually in color, but do not have to be.
- **Line drawings** are less detailed than pictures, and they are always in black and white.
- **Alpha-numeric symbols** are numbers and single letters.
- **Text** refers to full words, such as an index card with *c-e-r-e-a-l* on it.

These seven ways of depicting symbols can all be effective, depending on the situation, but they share one important drawback—they are all highly noun-oriented. It is very difficult to express verbs, prepositions, and adjectives with these types of symbols. Two additional types of visual symbols—static scene cues and dynamic scene cues—can be used to offset this weakness.

- **Static scene cues** combine visual symbols (usually photographs) often with a simultaneous spoken phrase. For example, the concept of a child's father arriving soon from work might be depicted with a picture of a man driving a car. As the child views the picture, the child's mother says, "Daddy is on his way home."
- **Dynamic scene** use computer technology or video to depict the action within a scene. For example, with a mouse click, an image of a boy may begin to walk down a sidewalk, past mailboxes, cars, pets, and so forth.

In the following chapter we provide a comprehensive description of static and dynamic scene cues and in Chapter 6 we show how different symbol levels can best be used to benefit learners with ASD.

comprehension and expression. For some, the difficulty lies with interpreting the message itself. For others, factors such as the length of the spoken sentence or rate at which it is delivered are the underlying cause of the misunderstanding.

Graphic Symbols (Print or Text)

Letters from our alphabet are graphic symbols that combine to form words in print that represent nouns, verbs, adverbs, adjectives, and so forth, which come together to represent broader ideas and concepts. To effectively use print, learners need to understand conceptually that written symbols represent the sounds that make up words, and then develop skills for identifying these written symbols.

Children acquire reading skills in a number of ways. A child's earliest understanding of print as a way to represent a known item is often through the identification of familiar logos, such as McDonald's, Toys R Us, or Dunkin Donuts. Some learners develop an extensive "sight word" vocabulary through repeated exposure to words that occur in a context, and then apply the patterns they learn in these words to novel words. For example, a child might learn the word "toys" from the store logo and then recognize the word "boys" when he sees it in a book. More commonly, learners learn to read through a phonics approach in which they gradually connect sounds with letters or groups of letters.

How well an individual with ASD uses graphic symbols depends on his particular strengths and weaknesses. Some have a strong aptitude; for example, many learners with ASD show strong interest in the credits of movies, and they often would rather flip through text-heavy books than play games or go to the playground. Others have less interest in graphic symbols. Often learners with autism perform better with written language because the coding of the information is not as transient as it is in spoken language (Shane & Simmons, 2001).

Perceptual Versus Semantic Understanding

A person's ability to communicate depends on how well he processes the gestural, visual, spoken, and graphic symbols he encounters. The key here is on which of two levels he understands these symbols. The first and most basic level is perceptual understanding—recognizing the symbol's outward characteristics. For example, a learner might:

- see an electrical device and perceive certain qualities, such as its size, shape, and color
- see a symbol and perceive it as a series of lines intersecting at different angles
- hear a word and perceive it as a series of sounds without meaning

Clearly, with only perceptual understanding, a symbol is of limited use. It is merely an isolated representation that carries little or no meaning. It does not truly become a symbol until the learner understands what it stands for. This more advanced level is known as semantic understanding—recognizing the symbol's larger meaning. Seeing an electrical device and recognizing it as a toaster, seeing a symbol and recognizing it as the letter "H," and hearing the word "challenge" and knowing its meaning demonstrate semantic understanding.

The phenomenon known as hyperlexia (also known an "empty reading") is a good example of the distinction between perceptual and semantic understanding. With hyperlexia, a person is capable of skillfully reading a text aloud, but does not understand the text's meaning. Learners with ASD often exhibit aspects of hyperlexia, that is, their ability to decode graphic symbols outpaces their ability to comprehend their meaning (Aram & Healy, 1988; Rimland, 1978). The label of hyperlexia is generally assigned when a child learns to decode on his own before age 3; in some cases, the child may have an obsessive attraction to text.

When instructing learners with autism, it is critical to consider whether they have perceptual or semantic understanding of a particular symbol. Often, they may have difficulty with semantic understanding because they lack the skills that would enable them to recognize unfamiliar symbols and understand their meaning. As a result, they may feel like they are being bombarded by hundreds of hard-to-decipher symbols. It is easy to understand how overwhelming and frustrating this can be.

For a symbol to promote semantic understanding, it must activate knowledge about the meaning associated with that symbol. In other words, the symbol triggers associations to specific referents, as well as previous knowledge associated with the referent. For example, a plane symbol on a highway sign alerts the driver to the concept of "airport" and activates prior knowledge and experiences associated with airports. The individual retrieves knowledge that this is a place where a person is required to go through a number of procedures to board a plane and travel to a new destination.

Effective symbol comprehension allows a person to achieve what is known as "stimulus equivalence"—treating symbols with different perceptual characteristics equally. In other words, the person successfully relates the visual symbol of a plane to the spoken word "plane" as well as the written word. This ease between symbol equivalency facilitates activating knowledge of the actual airport experience. The symbol is not a discrete entity intended to be an identical match to a specific airport (e.g., JFK or Heathrow), but a way to retrieve knowledge of the overall experience of airports. In terms of basic symbols used when working with individuals with ASD, a symbol of a pencil does not refer to a specific pencil the learner owns or has used; it serves as a way to retrieve knowledge of the pencil as part of a larger class of writing instruments and the experience of putting pencil to paper.

This ability to recognize unifying features within classes is vital because it enables a person to generalize—perceive the similarities between different stimuli (words, colors, sounds, lights, concepts, feelings, characteristics, and so forth). Without it, a person would see photos of a poodle, a Labrador retriever, and a pit bull and not recognize these within the larger classification of dogs. The ability to generalize experience leads to language growth.

Language Fundamentals

We now look at some key aspects of language that enable learners to derive meaning from symbols and develop the ability to speak, read, and write and generally communicate.

Semantics

Although semantic understanding refers to the broad concept of comprehending the larger meaning of something, "semantics" by itself usually refers to the many potential shades of meaning expressed in spoken or written language, depending on how a word or phrase is used. For example, in the sentence, "Someday I'd like to get a dog," the word "dog" has a broad categorical meaning (a four-legged animal that has fur and barks). In contrast, in the sentence, "Your dog destroyed my lawn," the word "dog" carries very specific meaning (such as a black Rottweiler named Max). A person's familiarity with particular words and how they are used together influences whether he understands the meaning of a particular phrase or sentence. When there is semantic understanding, words are bound to their meaning and the experience associated with them.

Individuals with ASD often have difficulty with semantics; they may encounter related words or phrases but fail to recognize they have the same meaning. For example, a child may know the phrase "no running in the hall," but fail to understand a teacher who states, "running is not allowed here."

Schema

Schema refers to the experiential knowledge we use to organize current knowledge and provide a framework for understanding. Examples of experiential knowledge include background knowledge, event knowledge, and procedural knowledge.

Background knowledge is the information we bring to a situation that can help us become oriented. For example, a teenager's prior knowledge of movie theaters allows

him to navigate his way through the process of buying a ticket and finding a seat, even if it is his first time at a particular theater. Having background knowledge reduces anxiety about entering into and competently navigating new situations.

Event knowledge refers to what we know about how to act at specific events. For example, a child learns that a birthday party includes certain rituals, such as the birthday child opening presents while others sing "Happy Birthday."

Procedural knowledge refers to our understanding of the function of the items within our environment and how to perform needed functions, such as tying our shoes or making a bowl of cereal.

Schema helps learners interpret symbols and, more broadly, organize and understand their world. Those with ASD often have difficulty summoning background and event knowledge. This can make adjustment to social situations difficult, especially if the setting is slightly different from a previous situation. For example, a child who has already attended several birthday parties may still try to open another child's presents or become disoriented by all the commotion of group play.

However, learners with ASD often have strong experiential knowledge skills. Through careful observation and trial and error, they may do exceptionally well at figuring out how to work mechanical devices (VCR, microwave, etc.) and assemble multipart devices from visually oriented instructions—without knowing the names of the pieces or being able to describe the functions of the devices they are handling. Such procedural skills seem to be attained without the aid of language.

Morphology

Morphology refers to the patterns of word structure in a particular language. For example, one word may have numerous endings, each of which affects its meaning. A reader of English recognizes that the words "books," "booklet," and "bookkeeper" all relate to the word "book," but have different meanings. Similarly, the words "rain," "rained," and "raining" are related but have different implications, as do "cats" and cat's."

Interpreting words' morphology is a major challenge for learners with ASD, which can make it hard for them to see connections between related words and determine whether a speaker is referring to the past, the present, or the future.

Syntax

Syntax refers to the rules that govern the way words combine to form phrases and phrases combine to form sentences. Each language has its own syntax, which determines factors such as word order, sentence organization, and the relationship between nouns and verbs. For example, in English one says, "I miss you," whereas in French one says, "tu me manque" (literally "you are missed by me").

Children gradually learn syntax by frequent exposure to conversation and participation in contextually based activities. The many variations in a language's syntax are not always logical. For exam-ple, in the sentence "before you eat, wash your hands," the order of events does not unfold in the order that they are mentioned. This contradiction between the linear arrangement of words in a sentence and the temporal ordering of the events they refer to can contribute to the difficulties individuals with ASD have in developing verbal skills.

Parts of Speech

The four most commonly used parts of speech for learners in the VIP Program are nouns, action verbs, prepositions, and adjectives.

Nouns

The most common way to think of a noun is as a word that refers to a person, place, thing, event, substance, or quality. The term derives from Latin *nomen* meaning name. Nouns can be classified in different ways, such as common nouns ("girl"), proper nouns ("Laura"), or collective nouns ("bunch," "herd"). Nouns can be substituted by pronouns ("she").

There is little doubt from both a clinical and research perspective that learners with ASD recognize nouns much more easily than other parts of speech. This recognition factor, which holds true whether the noun is represented in a spoken, graphic or written form, probably results from nouns usually referring to concrete items that can be felt, smelled, or tasted. A noun's concreteness makes it a good candidate to be touched, reproduced through a photograph or drawing, or represented by a physical model.

Because nouns can serve as the subject or object of a verb, learners with

ASD tend to recognize and comprehend the words that reside on both sides of the verb. For example, in the sentence, "David pushes the truck," a learner may know (or can often be easily taught) the proper noun David and recognize the common noun truck.

Action Verbs

Action verbs are words that denote an action or a state in which action refers to physical movement or activity. Learners with ASD tend to have difficulty understanding spoken, graphic, and text-based representations of verbs. Difficulty with the meaning of visuals intended to symbolize verbs, is most likely due to the inherent difficulty of portraying movement with a static representation. Because a static image cannot completely

capture or portray action, the action needs to be imagined. For example, a sentence that involves David acting on the truck (such as "Can you put David next to the truck?") may leave the learner at a loss if he is unsure of what "put" means in this context.

Because nouns and action verbs are the building blocks of speech, Table 2–1 highlights the differences in how easily they are portrayed with visual symbols. In Chapter 6, we offer strategies for overcoming barriers to comprehension of visual images of verbs.

Prepositions

A preposition is any member of a class of words used before nouns or pronouns to form phrases functioning as modifiers of verbs, nouns, or adjectives, and that

Table 2–1. Differences in How Easily Nouns and Verbs Are Portrayed with Visual Symbols

Nouns	Action Verbs
Concrete; has physical properties	More abstract; describes physical state, but does not have physical properties
Stands alone	Occurs in relation to an actor or object
Easy to determine the referent	Referent not as easily depicted
Tangible	Only becomes tangible in relation to a specific activity
Often child-directed (requesting)	Often adult-directed (instructing)
Often has an inherent reward (receiving a desired object)	Often has a secondary reward (pleasing an adult)
More easily represented; static images often effective	Less easily represented, static images often ineffective
Nontemporal	Temporal
Iconicity captures the essence of the image	Iconicity captures the essence of the movement

typically express a spatial, temporal, or other relationship. With prepositions, the spatial relationship of one feature to the totality of a graphic image is paramount. To effectively portray a preposition through visual representation, the graphic needs to contain two distinct elements that have a distinct relationship to each other. Accordingly, a smudge within a square and a dot within a circle can both stand for the preposition "in" as long as one recognizes that the smudge or dot is located inside the outer boundary. However, if the dot or smudge is merely seen as an independent mark, the relationship is lost and the concept is not conveyed.

Individuals with autism typically have difficulty with prepositions, as they do with many relational aspects of language. Prepositions can be especially confusing because spatial relationships may depend on the observer's perspective as well as the message's intent. For example, a book may be simultaneously on a table, beside a telephone, and under a lamp.

Adjectives

An adjective modifies a noun or a pronoun by describing, identifying, or quantifying words. Adjectives are essentially descriptors that are dependent on their referent to fully convey meaning. They are ambiguous until combined with a referent; the sentences "look at the red" and "it's a big" without the referent (such as a ball) carry little meaning.

For an individual to appreciate that a concept can be represented by some graphic image, some actual experience with the concept is essential. In other words, before one can appreciate that an image can relate to the idea of "wet" or "rough," familiarity with wetness and roughness must precede the introduc-

tion of the symbol meant to represent those ideas.

An adjective usually precedes the noun or the pronoun that it modifies. However, it is important to recognize that the adjective and its referent conceptually combine into one entity. The redness of the ball does not precede it; the ball is at once red.

The learner must appreciate the relationship between the adjective and the noun or pronoun to comprehend the intended message. Again, the persistent, confounding factor for individuals with ASD is in understanding the relational aspects of language, in this case between the descriptor and its referent.

Adjectives that describe states of being (feelings) can be especially problematic. For example, one can depict the sentence "Laura is a happy girl" with a girl's happy face and the sentence "Greg felt sick" with a boy's sad face or someone holding his stomach. A learner with an effective schematic or experiential background can associate the facial expression to prior experience and make the symbolic connection, and thus see the relationship between the symbol and the feeling. Learners with ASD often have trouble comprehending these states of being, as well as the terms used to describe such states.

Phonology

Phonology refers to the way sounds function within a language. Awareness of a language's phonology allows us to divide sentences into words and words into syllables. Early in their development of phonological awareness, toddlers perceive a sentence such as "I want a cookie" as one long word ("Iwannacookie"). Being able to break it into separate sounds, syllables, and words is a key step in learning to use language, as it enables learners to generate new sentences with similar constructions, such as "I want juice" and "Do you want a cookie?" Moreover, developing awareness of the sounds within words is a critical step in reading and spelling acquisition. Phonological awareness is another area in which learners with ASD often trail behind typically developing learners.

Use

Use refers to how language is applied in different contexts to convey an intended meaning. Use may also be referred to as pragmatics. Uses of language include greeting and parting ("Hello"), requesting ("I want pizza"), protesting ("Leave me alone"), and commenting ("I like your coat"). Commenting is especially important because it is the key to advanced social interaction. There are several types of commenting:

Commenting on topics of interest to oneself. This form of commenting is self-directed and includes topics such as a person's daily activities, personal anecdotes, and events in the immediate environment that capture one's attention. To engage in this type of commenting, a person needs to only initiate conversation with another person.

Commenting on topics of interest to others. This requires knowledge or inferred knowledge of another's interests. In addition to initiating conversation, this type of commenting requires the ability to take turns, maintain the conversation, correct any mistaken assumptions (what is known as conversational repairs), and request clarification.

Commenting on topics of shared interest to both communication partners. This includes social gratuities such as greetings and partings, as well as comments on the weather, food, entertainment, leisure, gossip, and so forth. Along with the skills required for commenting on topics of interest to others, commenting on topics of shared interest requires the ability to change topics.

Learners with ASD often use language for greeting, requesting, and protesting, but they may have difficulty with commenting, especially commenting on topics of interest to others and of shared interest, which requires taking the perspective of another.

Discourse

Discourse refers to any unit of connected speech or writing longer than a sentence. Discourse allows a person to construct longer descriptions and explanations. It can be used for two broad purposes: narrative and exposition.

Narrative refers to a story; to understand a narrative discourse a person must keep track of elements such as characters, settings, and events. We use narrative to tell the events of our lives; who we saw, where we were, when things occurred, how we responded, and what the outcome was.

Exposition is intended to convey or explain information; often it is described as a main idea and supporting detail. To understand expository discourse, a person must follow the explanation of a process, which frequently has multiple steps, and understand the relationship of these steps to completion of a final goal. The steps in getting prepared to go off to school or for brushing one's teeth typically follow an expository form.

Typically developing children practice their narrative skills by telling the autobiographical story of their days. Children with ASD generally lag behind in their ability to use narrative discourse, including skills such as labeling events, sequencing events, and identifying the causal relationship between events. Their use of expository discourse may be hindered by a reduced ability to perceive the main idea (whole concept) and supporting detail (steps in the process).

As we have seen, individuals with ASD have difficulty with many of the fundamentals of language acquisition, but may have real strengths in certain areas. In the next chapter, we describe in detail how the three modes of the Visual Immersion Program can be used to address their specific needs.

References

Aram, D. M., & Healy, J. F. (1988). Hyperlexia: A review of extraordinary word recognition. In L. K. Obler & D. Fein (Eds), *The exceptional brain: Neuropsychology of talent and special ability* (pp. 70–102). New York: Guilford Press.

Rimland, B. (1978). Savant capabilities of autistic children and their cognitive implications. In G. Serban (Ed.), *Cognitive defects in the development of mental illness* (pp. 43–65). New York: Brunner/Mazel.

Shane, H. C., & Simmons, M. (2001, November). *The use of visual supports to enhance communication and improve problem behaviors.* Paper presented at the annual meeting of the American Speech-Language-Hearing Association, New Orleans, LA.

Wetherby, A., & Prizant, B. (2000). *Autism spectrum disorders: A transactional developmental perspective.* Baltimore: Paul H. Brookes.

Wetherby, A. M., Prizant, B. M., & Hutchinson, T. (1998). Communicative, social affective, and symbolic profiles of young children with autism and developmental disorder. *American Journal of Speech-Language Pathology, 7*, 79–91.

3

Presenting Visuals in the Three Modes of the VIP

The use of visual symbols to help learners with ASD improve their communication skills has been an important component of clinical work since the 1980s. However, symbols are often applied inconsistently and without an overall approach. A systematic application of visuals with a prescribed scope and sequence based on the learner's strengths and weaknesses is more likely to lead to increased comprehension, speech production, language growth, and overall improvement in behavior.

Our program offers a comprehensive model based on using visuals in three modes—expression, instruction, and organization. The three modes use a range of visual symbols in a variety of ways. Before examining the modes themselves, we first need to review the ways visual symbols can be presented and the types of communication displays in which they are used.

Visual Cues

Visual symbols can be presented in two ways, as element cues or scene cues.

Element Cues

An element cue is a symbol that illustrates an individual component within a scene. There are six types used within VIP:

- **Agent element cues**—symbols that represent people or characters (conventionally referred to as nouns)
- **Object element cues**—symbols that represent things that can be seen, touched, or heard (also nouns)
- **Action element cues**—symbols that represent activity (verbs)

- **Spatial element cues**—symbols that indicate the position of one object with respect to another (prepositions)
- **Attribute element cues**—symbols that describe a key quality or characteristic of an agent, action, or object (adjectives)
- **Temporal element cues**—symbols that indicate duration or frequency (generally are adjectives or adverbs).

Figure 3–1 provides examples of the different types of element cues.

Element cues can be presented singly or in combined form. For example, a picture of a dog (an agent element cue) is a single element cue. A picture of a dog presented simultaneously with a picture of a brown circle (attribute element cue) and a picture of legs running (action element cue) is a combined element cue that represents a brown dog running. Combined element cues provide detailed information about a situation or event, but require greater understanding of semantic relationships from the learner.

Scene Cues

A scene cue is a single photograph that portrays a concept or a command. For example, pointing to a picture of a boy kicking a ball while saying "he kicks the ball" portrays the concept of a ball-kicking, and holding up a picture of a learner wearing his coat and saying "get your coat" communicates this directive. A scene cue is intended to visually capture a spoken message's essence or intent; it is not an exact picture-for-word match to the spoken message, but an opportunity to process information as a whole (e.g., gestalt).

There are two types of scene cues: static and dynamic.

1. **Static scene cues.** A static scene cue uses an image or images that do not move, such as photos or drawings. There are two types of scene cues: "premade" and "buildable." A premade scene cue is one in which a single image presents

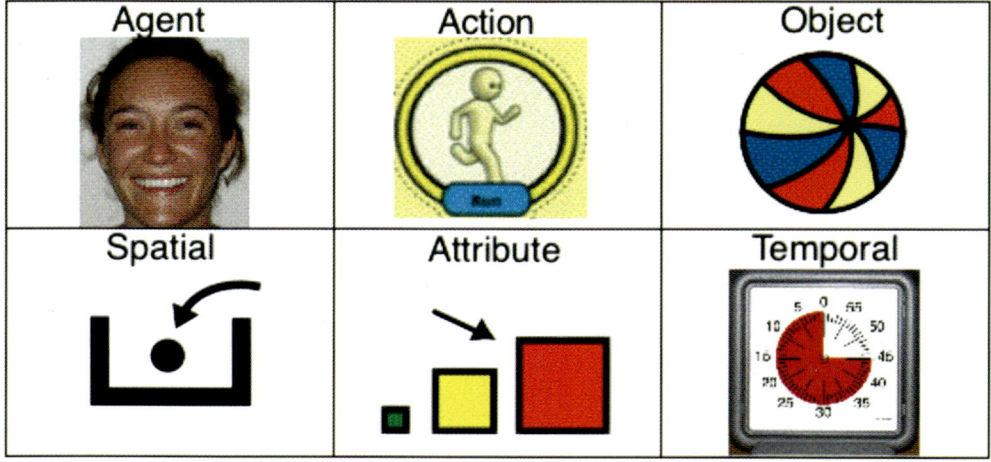

Figure 3–1. Examples of six types of element cues. (From The Picture Communication Symbols ©1981–2007 by Mayer-Johnson LLC. All Rights Reserved Worldwide. Used with permission.)

the entire scene, such as a picture of a boy riding a horse. A buildable scene cue combines more than one image to create a small scene. For example, separate pictures of a horse and a boy positioned in relation to each other against a backgound combine to represent the scene of a boy riding a horse.

2. **Dynamic scene cues.** A dynamic scene cue uses an image that moves, such as an animated cartoon character that is running on a computer display, a video clip of a person running, or a toy figurine that can be manipulated by the learner or the instructor. For example, the instructor can sit down at a table with a flexible toy character, a car, a truck, and a block (Figure 3–2). To build the association between the visual scene and the action it represents, the instructor can say, "the boy pushes the truck," "the boy climbs the ladder," and "the boy jumps on the block" as the instructor demonstrates these maneuvers.

As the learner becomes accustomed to seeing visuals in a relevant context and in combination with speech, scene cues can be incorporated into daily life. At home, parents can take snapshots of commonly used items and then present these pictures at appropriate times. For example, a child's mother might hold up a picture of the learner wearing his jacket as she says, "Time to get your jacket," and then show a picture of the family in the car as she says "Let's get into Mommy's car." Although it is not possible to have a visual for everything the child does, this technique is feasible and effective when parents focus on the actions related to the most common daily activities (such as getting ready for school, meals, and bedtime).

Communication Displays

Element cues and scene cues provide the content that fills in the target areas of the various communication displays

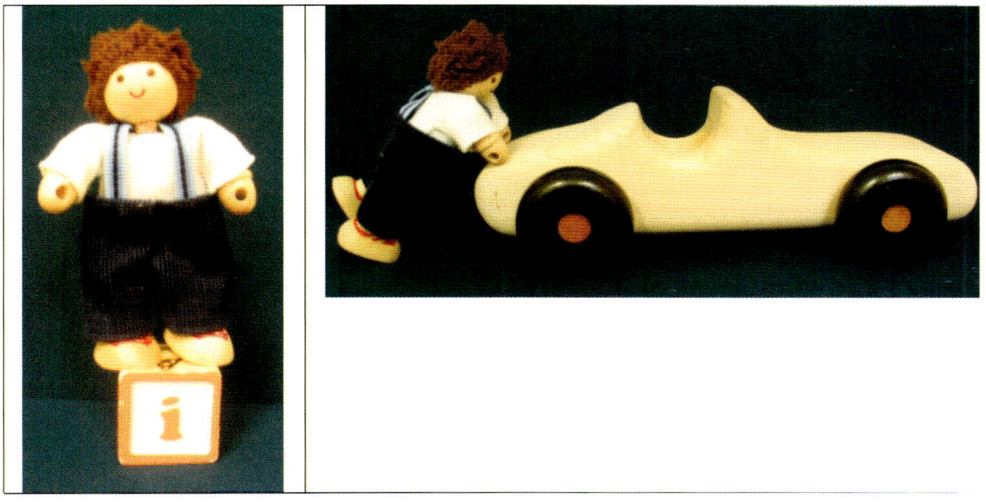

Figure 3–2. Examples of scene cues representing (1) Boy on block and (2) Boy push car.

instructors and parents use when working with learners with ASD. There are three types of displays: grid displays, whole scene displays, and mixed displays.

Grid Displays

The most common type of visual display features a grid format, that is, a blank background onto which the learner can place visual symbols, which typically ends up having a gridlike appearance. Most commonly, the grid is made of heavy paper or cardboard, and Velcro is typically used so the visual cues can be affixed to and removed from the grid. A computer screen also can function as a grid, often allowing for multiple pages; we will discuss computer displays in detail in Chapter 6. Common types of grid displays include:

Communication Book Displays

The grid format is used in communication books, which are notebooks containing graphic symbols. The first published descriptions of a communication book display format were designed to be used by learners with cerebral palsy who experienced limited or lack of speech (Goldberg & Fenton, n.d.; McDonald & Schultz, 1973; Vicker, 1974). The most well-known form of communication book display used by people with ASD is a PECS book (Frost & Bondy, 1994) that in use typically depicts preferred nouns representing desired items. The one difference between the original communication books and those used in the PECS program is a strip of removable Velcro on the cover of the book to which a learner places visual cues before handing the strip to the listener.

Conversation Displays

Grids can be used to display a series of symbols arranged by grammatical category that all relate to a single topic of particular interest to the learner, such as a favorite sports activity, his preferred games, information about a group of animals, or preparation of a favorite food. A "message window" is placed above the grid onto which visuals are affixed. For example, a grid display about preparing a pizza might include visuals of flour, tomato sauce, cheese, people involved in the preparation, utensils such as spoons and knives, and action verbs such as cutting, pouring, and baking (Figure 3–3). Conversation displays are used to aid comprehension as well as to assist in expression.

Conversation displays also can be used to remind the learner of a prior experience or direct him to carry out an activity. For example, an agent element cue of a picture of "Grandma" activates the experience of getting in the car, driving to Grandma's house, and the anticipated experience at Grandma's house. Combined action/object element cues such as the symbols for "drink + milk" can be used to direct the learner to pour himself a glass of milk.

Note that conversation displays are processed analytically—that is, the learner views each element one at a time and gradually gains meaning from the larger display based on his understanding of the semantic relationships between each element. Such analytic processing represents the beginning of the learner's ability to generate a visual language system.

An important aspect of grid displays is that the initial grid is "decontextualized"—the display is out of the context in which it occurs. The learner begins

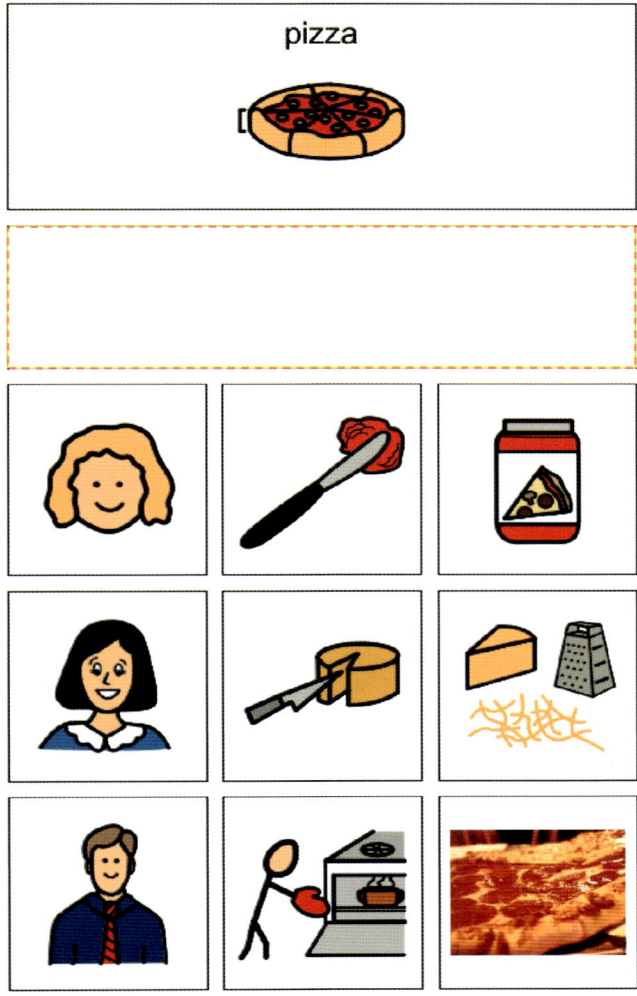

Figure 3–3. Example of a conversational display using multiple agents for preparing pizza. (From The Picture Communication Symbols ©1981–2007 by Mayer-Johnson LLC. All Rights Reserved Worldwide. Used with permission.)

with a blank slate, and the display gains meaning as items are added. In some cases, beginning with a decontextualized display may be advantageous, as it provides an open-ended forum for the learner to explore what he is most interested in. With conversational displays, the instruc-

tor should use whatever type of visual support the learner is most comfortable with, either from a communication book or from other sources, such as snapshots or pictures clipped from magazines. If possible, it is helpful to have some of the actual items available. To lay the basis for broad use of language, the instructor should ask a variety of questions that will elicit many types of responses, such as: What is your favorite food? Who in your family likes ice cream? Which food did you eat yesterday?

If the learner requests a cookie, the instructor can expand the dialogue by asking if, for example, he wants to share the cookie. So ideally, instead of just saying, "I want a cookie," the individual learns sentences that use a variety of subjects, verbs, and objects, such as, "You're eating the cookie," and "I gave you a snack."

Use of conversation displays dates back to the 1940s, when Edith Fitzgerald proposed using them to help deaf children learn language structure and communicate (Fitzgerald, 1949. In Chapter 6, we provide greater detail on the creation of conversation displays.

Visual Schedules

Grids can be used to create a personalized daily schedule that lays out sequentially the important events of a learner's day (Figure 3–4). Visual symbols such as photographs, pictures, and text are arranged vertically or horizontally (MacDuff et al., 1993; Pierce & Schreibman, 1994). A similar display format can be used to outline a series of events or steps within a given activity, such as a class at school, a meeting with an instructor, or a birthday party. A more comprehensive description of the design and application of visual schedules is provided in Chapter 6.

Temporal Displays

Temporal displays help the learner understand time-related aspects of learning, such as how much time has elapsed, how

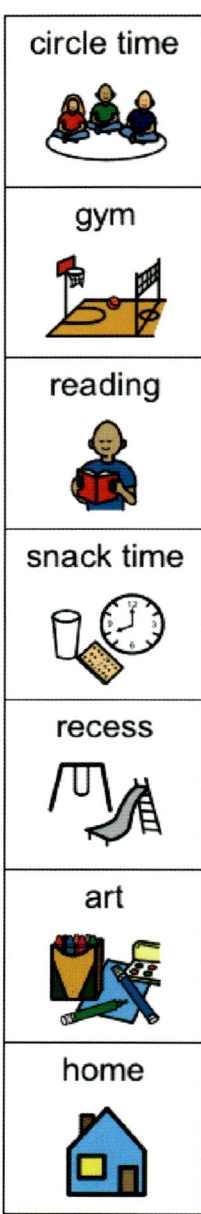

Figure 3–4. Example of a typical visual schedule. (From The Picture Communication Symbols ©1981–2007 by Mayer-Johnson LLC. All Rights Reserved Worldwide. Used with permission.)

many trials are needed to complete a task, and what the reinforcement for a specified activity is. Examples include:

- Visual timers, such as the Time Timer™, stopwatches, and hourglass timers
- First/then displays, such as a tabletop display that shows a visual representing a first activity (often the task) on the left side and a visual representing the follow-up activity (often the reward) on the right side. Chapter 6 provides greater detail on creating effective first/then displays.
- Countdown displays, such as boards with tokens removed each time the learner accomplishes a task, subtractive finger countdowns (such as the instructor holding up his hand and counting down each time the learner accomplishes a task), and reward

displays (such as the instructor presenting 10 pistachio nuts and allowing the learner to eat one for every correct answer).

Whole Scene Displays

Whole scene displays (also known as visual scene displays, or VSDs) provide a panoramic view of a large background. This enables the learner to portray events, people, actions, objects, and activities in the context within which they occur or exist. They can represent a generic context (e.g., a kitchen, a house with yard, or a school room with a teacher and students) or a personalized context (e.g., the view from a specific child's bedroom [Figure 3–5] or the view of a place he enjoys visiting, such as relative's house, the zoo, etc.).

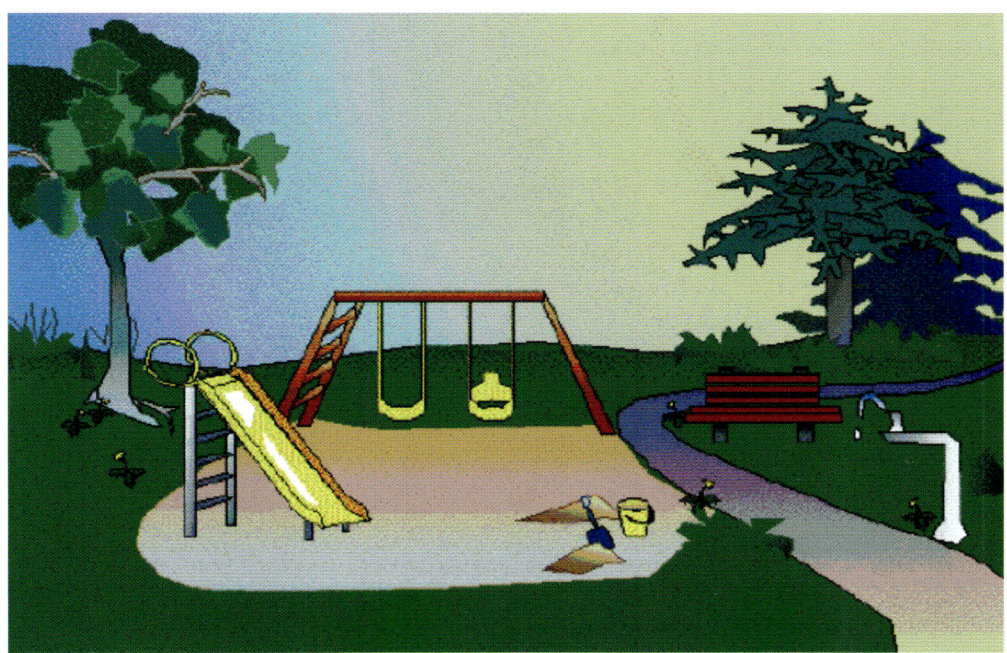

Figure 3–5. Example of a whole scene display (playground).

Typically, a large photograph is used to depict the whole scene, and relevant objects can be added to the background by using Velcro. Computer screens also can be used; clicking on a "hot spot" in the background temporarily displays a larger picture.

As with scene cues, whole scenes can be "premade" or "buildable." With a premade whole scene, the panoramic view already includes the key elements within it (i.e., a kitchen that includes the refrigerator, the stove, a microwave oven, a table, etc.). The learner can point out objects, place cut-outs on top of similar or identical objects, and add additional elements to the scene. With a buildable whole scene, the panoramic view is basically a background and the learner builds the scene by adding elements such as people or objects into it.

Whole scene displays can consist of a single scene that makes up the entire display, or multiple scenes on a page that reflect the place of occurrence, event, or sequence of the steps in a routine. To work with a whole scene, the learner and the instructor can sit at a table with the scene background displayed in front of them, along with relevant visual images. Visuals accompanying a whole scene depicting the view from the bedroom window might include a car, a squirrel, a dog, a ball, a snowman, a mailman, and other pedestrians. The instructor begins by asking a broad question, such as "What do you see outside your window," and lets the learner's answers guide the direction of the ensuing exchange.

In addition to skills the learner uses with conversation displays, whole scenes encourage expanded use of language, including greater use of verbs. For example, if the learner's answer to the initial question is "I see a car," the instructor can encourage him to use "car" in sentences involving verbs such as "go," "park," and "drive." As with grid displays, the instructor can ask the learner to act out some of the activities inspired by the scene. Questions such as, "Where do you kick the ball?" might lead to an exchange about balls, and the learner can be encouraged to say, "I kick the ball" as he does so in the room.

Whole scenes are an especially effective way to promote a learner's ability to communicate, for three reasons:

- Whereas traditional picture books use images of isolated nouns to depict a person (*who*), place (*where*), or object (*what*) in isolation, whole scenes can convey all these themes simultaneously.
- Whole scenes are likely to provide greater meaning of schematic or experiential content to learners with ASD, including those who may not comprehend the semantic meaning behind images of isolated nouns.
- Whole scenes are particularly appealing to young children because they are realistic and personal, and their interactive nature tends to lead to enjoyable, engaging conversations. Light et al. (2006) reported that children 3 to 4 years of age had greater proficiency with information represented by a visual scene display than through a more traditional grid display with a more decontexualized symbol content.

Note that whole scenes are contextualized and processed as a unified whole (gestalt). The learner relies on the embedded context within the scene to glean meaning from it (Light et al., 2004).

Mixed Displays

Visual information can also be presented in ways that combine aspects of grid and scene displays. Such mixed displays can be used as a transitional bridge between contextualized whole scenes and analytical conversation displays. For example, elements that describe the scene can be entered into a message window under the scene, as in Figure 3–6. Such a display combines analytical processing with

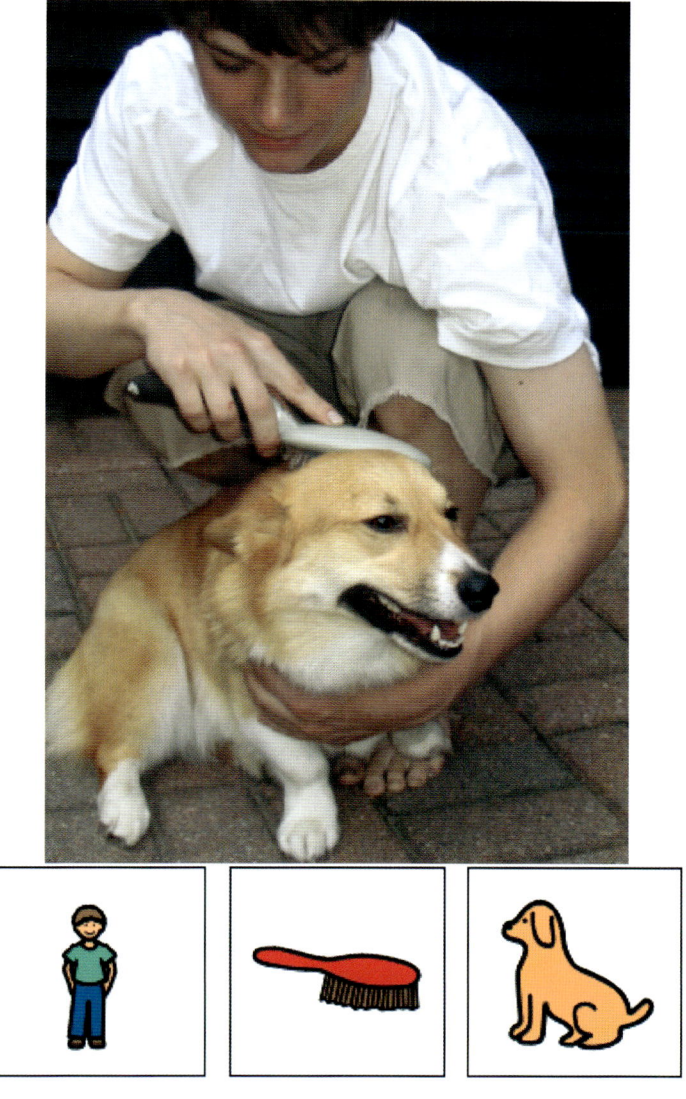

Figure 3–6. Mixed scene display depicting "boy brushes dog." (From The Picture Communication Symbols ©1981–2007 by Mayer-Johnson LLC. All Rights Reserved Worldwide. Used with permission.)

gestalt processing, providing a structured method for gradually moving the learner from using whole scenes to using conversation displays.

The Three Modes

We now examine the three modes of the VIP and how the tools we have just covered can be used in these modes.

Visual Expressive Mode (VEM)

The first mode of the Visual Immersion Program involves using a full complement of visual resources for purposes of expressive communication. In the VEM, visual symbols such as line drawings, photographs, and entire visual scenes are used to express thoughts or ideas. The symbols may supplement a spoken message or stand alone. A person can use the VEM to make requests (e.g., for food, a pen, television, etc.), comment on feelings and experiences, give or get information, construct and answer questions, and so on. In its broadest sense, the VEM is a tool for a person to tell the story of his life.

Note that the VEM is not unique to individuals with autism. To understand this mode, it may be helpful to take a moment to consider that in all human social interaction, the output is expressive, and this output can be expressed with all types of symbols (spoken, gestural, visual, and graphic). Anytime we use a symbol for expression along with a visual element, we are using the VEM. Common examples of the VEM that we encounter in everyday life include hand-written letters, E-mail, close-captioning on television, and the pictures and graphics used to support a newscaster's words.

The first reported use of visuals for expressive communication for individuals with ASD occurred in the early 1980s, with the recognition that children with ASD often have strong visual-spatial skills (Schuler & Baldwin, 1981). A host of visually based strategies followed, and using visuals for expression—especially for requesting desired goods and services—became a popular communication technique among parents, therapists and teachers who interact with individuals with autism. PECS, an innovation of the early 1990s, represents the most well-known example of using visuals to help learners with expression.

Using visuals to request items is highly effective because of the constant positive reinforcement inherent in the activity. The learner requests the items most important to him and then receives them, so once he learns to use visuals to make requests he is likely to continue doing so. This is an important first step. By making requests, the individual learns that symbols represent actual items, and he learns that he has the power to communicate.

It is important, however, to recognize that requesting is just a starting point in use of visuals for expression. Ideally, the learner should be able to do much more—to give and receive more detailed information, to ask questions, and to comment. In short, to engage in a conversation. Conversation displays, whole scenes, and scene cues can help learners express themselves more broadly.

Visual Instruction Mode (VIM)

The second mode of the VIP focuses on instruction—using visual elements (such as photos, objects, or gestures) as a substitute or complement for spoken or written language to enhance commands or directions.

The emphasis of the VIM is on building language comprehension, which we view as the foundation for acquiring and applying language. In many cases, the learner may actually be capable of literally acting on a spoken command, but cannot process its intent because the linguistic structure is too advanced (a comprehension deficit) or the command is spoken too fast (an auditory processing deficit).

The simultaneous and sustained presentation of a visual that illustrates the ephemeral spoken command offers the learner a better opportunity for comprehension than a series of discrete visual symbols. (See The Myth of a Visual Symbol Alignment below.)

Aspects of the VIM are used in several existing approaches, including aided language (Goossens et al., 1992), aided language stimulation (Dexter, 1998), augmented input (Mirenda & Erickson, 2000; Wood et al., 1998), partner augmented input (Romski & Sevcik, 1996),

The Myth of a Visual Symbol Alignment

When done improperly, constructing a statement or command from a series of visual images can create a confusing rather than clarifying experience. For example, mapping pictures to exact English word order can interfere with meaning because meaning comes across differently with discrete graphic symbols than it does through spoken words. What results is a string of disparate images whose meaning is largely impossible to decipher.

This phenomenon occurs because spoken language contains a rule-governed word order (syntax). A typically developing child learns this word order through repeated exposure to verbal communication during contextually based activities. Unfortunately, the rules of syntax do not directly transfer over to a display of visual symbols.

The problem is that constructing a sentence with a string of pictures focuses the child on the sentence's structure rather than meaning. For this technique to be effective, even for purely expressive purposes, the rule system regarding word order needs to be obvious and explicit to the learner.

Figure 3–A contains a set of pictures accompanied by English text for the sentence, "The boy pushes the girl who is sitting in the wagon." It is a perfectly coherent sentence in either spoken or written form because a rule-governed syntactic order with a specific semantic intent has been applied. A person who can read would have no trouble understanding the written words, and could match up the pictures to the relevant text.

However, consider what Figure 3–A conveys to someone who cannot read. If we eliminate the text, the message is nearly impossible to interpret, because the visual symbols have no obvious relationship to each other. The string of symbols is a series of discrete pictures that are not tied together by a set of linguistic conventions, which normally would improve the likelihood of comprehension.

Figure 3–B uses a scene cue to convey the same information contained in Figure 3–A. Although this scene cue is not governed by rules or part of an actual language, visual or otherwise, it clearly conveys the message, demonstrating that a simple picture express a complete idea.

Too often, we as practitioners have used approaches that place a series of symbols in exact English word order which we have come to believe is an intuitive but ultimately misguided attempt to address a complex problem. PECS books, computer-based communication programs, and many other communication approaches for individuals with ASD use discrete symbol elements that do not connect one grammatical category with another. Rather, these approaches use a set of graphic symbols that have meaning in isolation (e.g., a symbol for a watch looks like and can stand for a watch) or as isolated units, but do not necessarily have a logical association or relationship when those discrete symbols are arranged in sequence.

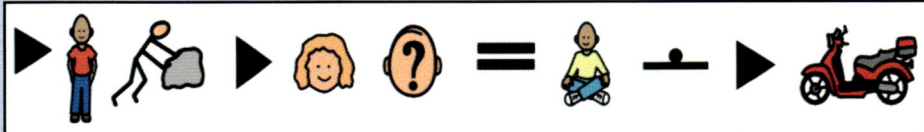

Figure 3–A. Example of one-to-one correspondence between visual symbols and spoken words in a sentence (to represent, "The boy pushes the girl who is sitting on the scooter.") (From The Picture Communication Symbols ©1981–2007 by Mayer-Johnson LLC. All Rights Reserved Worldwide. Used with permission.)

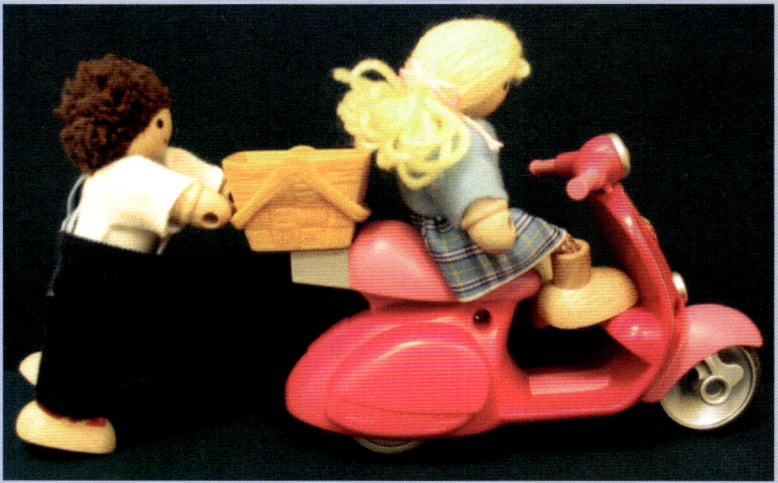

Figure 3–B. Example of whole scene representing, "The boy pushes the girl who is sitting on the scooter.")

and visually cued speech (Quill, 1995). These approaches tend to introduce symbols in an orderly manner, but the symbols are not typically presented in a way that makes language comprehension the primary focus.

Within the VIP scene cues are an essential component of the VIM. The advantage of scene cues is that they can represent a whole idea or complete thought through a single visual image. Eventually, the learner comes to understand what is portrayed in the scene cues: He understands the intention of the task by viewing the scene cue (generally accompanied by a spoken directive), and carries out the command.

From a developmental standpoint, scene cues serve two related purposes:

- They play a compensatory role, improving comprehension of a spoken message.
- They serve as a therapeutic tool to improve auditory comprehension, with the intention of gradually reducing dependence on the visual scene cue until a spoken message is understood on its own.

Because scene cues establish the link between a visual scene and the activity it represents, they are especially helpful for learners with ASD who are able to sort and match pictures and objects and can recognize nouns (characters) but have difficulty interpreting relational language (e.g., prepositions, action verbs). This disparate ability to comprehend different grammatical categories is common among learners with autism.

Scene cues also are useful for teaching practical tasks such as tying one's shoes or making a snack. The instructor displays the appropriate scene cue ("First we put the right lace over the left lace," "Now we cut the sandwich in two pieces," etc.) as he or she demonstrates each step in the sequence of the task.

Recent research supports the use of scene cues: In numerous clinical trials where scenes cues were introduced, learners with ASD performed better when speech was combined with a scene than when speech was used alone (Shane & Douglas, 2002).

A key point about spoken language without accompanying visual support is that we often do not know which parts of the message the learner comprehends. He may understand all, part, or none of the spoken message, and all or part of the visual element. The important point is that combining the spoken and visual message is more effective than either component by itself. Exactly what percentage of information is understood through which avenue is less important than the goal of the learner understanding the overall intent of the message.

Note that the VEM and the VIM are often closely intertwined. A scene cue, for example, actually uses both modes. In making the statement, "Put the shoes in the closet" and displaying the visual, the instructor (the sender) is expressing information (use of the VEM). But from the perspective of the learner (the receiver), he is being instructed (use of the VIM).

The VIM and Sign Language

It should be pointed out that the VIM functions much like American Sign Language does for deaf individuals. Both communication methods do not rely on a literal word-for-word replication of spoken language. In other words, a sign language interpreter communicating the

---

Avoiding Unintended Interference to Comprehension Using Speech

In all three modes of VIP—and when working with learners with ASD in general—the instructor should avoid complex phrases and avoid rephrasing statements in a way that may confuse the learner.

This approach may run counter to the way adults often converse with typically developing individuals; if a toddler does not seem to understand what an adult says, the adult will often use different words to say the same thing. For example, a mother may hold up an apple and say, "Do you want an apple?" If the learner does not react, she may rephrase her question as, "Are you hungry—how about a snack?"

Although this technique is useful for typically developing children, it can make comprehension harder for individuals with ASD, who often take longer to process auditory information. As a result, rephrasing a question can have the unintended result of confusing the learner; as he attempts to process the words in the first phrase, a second sentence with different words arrives, and now all the words become jumbled, further muddying the sentence's meaning.

We refer to this phenomenon as "unintended interference to comprehension." To avoid it, we recommend repeating the identical phraseology, with sufficient pauses of several seconds between each attempt to give the learner who has a history of difficulty processing auditory information sufficient time to respond, before rephrasing the statement.

---

sentence "What time is your dentist appointment?" does not have six different signs for the words in this question, and an instructor using the VIM would not display six pictures to illustrate it.

Another similarity is that both communication methods may use multiple avenues of expression. A deaf person receives the information primarily from the speaker's hand signs, but may also get some information from other cues, such as reading lips and viewing the speaker's facial expressions. With the VIM, the learner has an opportunity to receive information from visual symbols in combination with spoken words.

Visual Organization Mode (VOM)

The final mode of the VIP is organization—using visual symbols to sequentially organize a task, activity, or schedule. Daily schedules and other time-oriented displays (timers, countdown displays, first-then displays) are common examples of the VOM, and this mode can also be used to depict the steps in a multipart task (such as making an omelet). A number of researchers have shown that visuals are effective for these purposes (Quill, 1995).

In all uses of the VOM, instructors should strive to give the learner as much information as possible and to be as specific as possible. It is important to provide greater detail than is typically given when a single symbol is meant to represent an event (Shane, 2006). This additional information serves to offer clarity and reduce anxiety or confusion about the impending event or activity. For example, before beginning a 15-minute class on making a sandwich, the instructor can show the learner a display breaking the class down into three 4-minute segments on say, gathering the ingredients, making a sandwich, and eating the sandwich, with a 3-minute segment at the end for cleaning up. The individuals involved in the activity can be highlighted, as well as the activity location. Similarly, if a learner is being asked to complete a drawing task, the instructor might create a first-then display showing that when the learner draws (the "first" portion of the display), he can play a computer game (the "then" portion of the display) (Figure 3–7A). The VIP expands on this concept, whereby the opportunity to play for 10 minutes and create four drawings is depicted (Figure 3–7B).

Note that the information conveyed here is beneficial even when dealing with unpleasant things. First, the learner knows that the work portion (drawing four pictures) has a definite end, so he is less likely to become bored or frustrated during the activity. Second, he knows the fun portion (the computer game) has a definite end, so he is less likely to become upset when the endpoint arrives.

Behavioral Benefits: Order from Chaos

Used in this fashion, the VOM is an effective tool for helping individuals with ASD

reduce confusion about the day's transitions and react to changes in their routine, minimizing anxiety and reducing both inward and outward aggression. It is not uncommon for a learner with autism to react negatively or even violently to changes in routine. A clear VOM serves as an alert about an impending transition and shows the learner what is about to happen. It can prevent a learner from being surprised when life's normal transitions unfold.

It is likely that the VOM leads to more socially appropriate behavior because behavior problems among individuals with ASD are often a secondary effect of a spoken language and information processing deficit. If a learner cannot comprehend basic spoken statements that mark transitions or denote abrupt and unexpected changes (e.g., "After you play the computer game for 10 minutes, you will have to go back to your regular class"), he has little way to know what is about to happen, and each event is a last-second surprise. The learner encounters similar time-oriented statements all day long ("Get your coat—we are going to Grammy's house," "Time to turn off the TV—it's time for dinner"), so it is vital that he learn to understand them.

Not having the ability to understand such instructions is a little like being awoken from the comfort of a sound sleep and moved to a new location. For the learner with a spoken language difficulty who is uncertain about the events of the day, this hasty awakening occurs constantly, making life a chaotic experience. Using the VOM to give a warning often has an immediate and positive effect on behavior, attitude, and learning.

The VOM also is an important tool for establishing routines and habits,

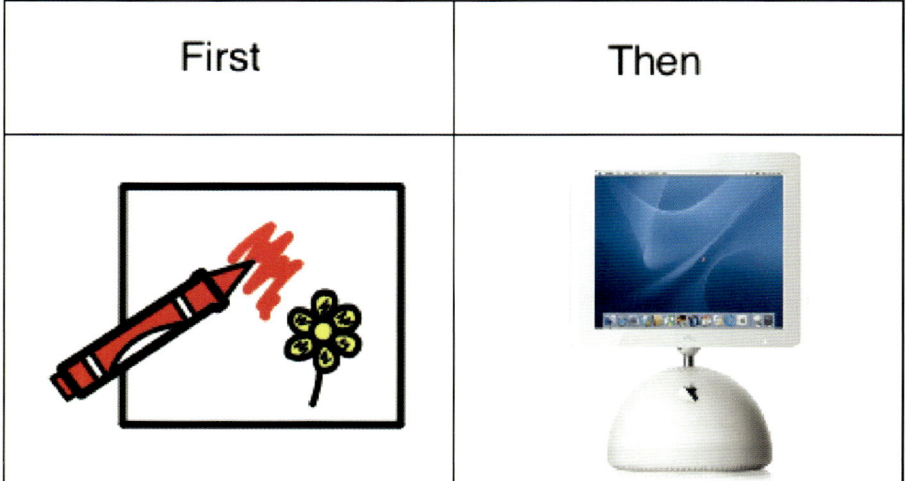

A.

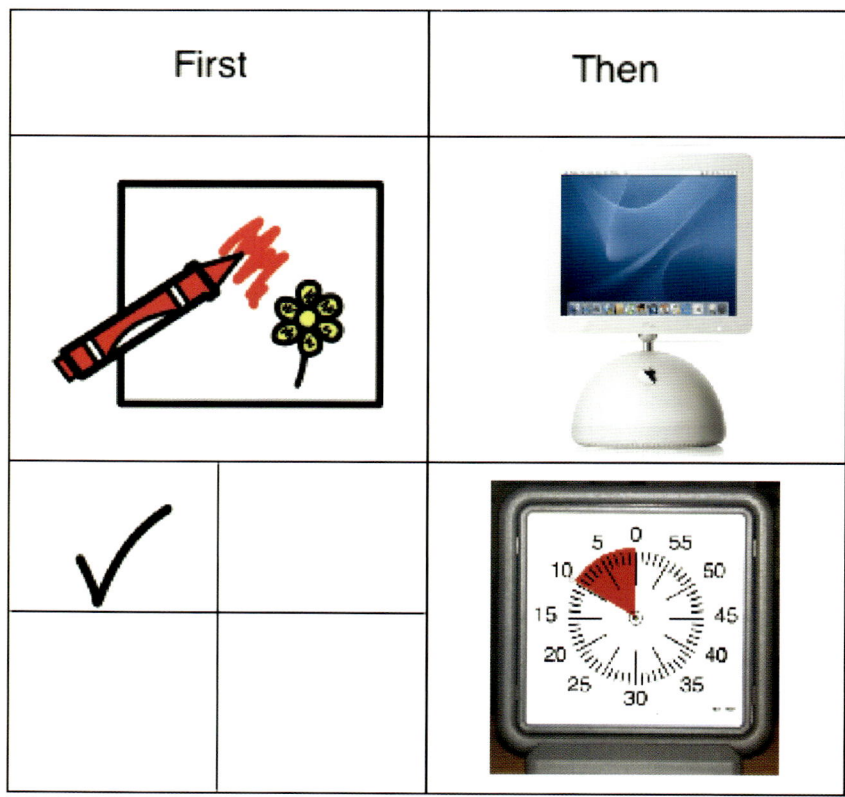

B.

Figure 3–7. **A.** Example of a typical first/then display (representing "first draw, then computer"). **B.** Example of an expanded first/then display (representing "first draw 4 pictures, then computer for 10 minutes"). (From The Picture Communication Symbols ©1981–2007 by Mayer-Johnson LLC. All Rights Reserved Worldwide. Used with permission.)

which people with ASD often find deeply comforting. The VOM can be used to create a display showing after-dinner activities, such as the individual getting to watch a video after he straightens up his room.

More broadly, the VOM plays a key role in laying the foundation for a more complex understanding of time. Comprehending that certain events have a causal relationship with other events helps the learner develop the ability to predict and infer what is going to happen based on prior experiences. This is critical for the learner to come to understand that rewards are not always immediate. For example, it is an important behavioral step when a learner can understand that if he behaves well for a month, he will get to go to a baseball game, or that if he completes certain household chores, he will get a monthly allowance.

Does Visual Language Enhance or Blunt Speech?

In practice, the VEM, the VOM, and the VIM are used together. Over time, the learner becomes comfortable using visual scene displays, visual schedules, scene cues, and other tools from the visual arsenal to communicate. This raises an important issue, which is sometimes voiced by parents and instructors: Does using visuals as the foundation for communication interfere with spoken language acquisition?

Based on our clinical experience, the answer is no. In fact, we believe just the opposite: We consider visuals an excellent form of speech therapy. We have worked with many individuals with ASD

who began speaking or made significant improvements in their speaking abilities after they learned to use visual language.

We do not know precisely why this is the case. Perhaps seeing visual images allows learners with ASD to better organize information and rehearse what they want to say. At a neurological level, perhaps visual language activates parts of the brain that were not previously used for communication (the phenomenon of "intersystemic reorganization") (Luria, 1980).

Regardless of the mechanism, the important point is that visual speech enhances rather than blunts the learner's ability to speak. We consider it analogous to crutches—people who break a leg only use crutches as long as they need to; they are anxious to start walking again as soon as possible. Similarly, individuals with ASD want to speak, and they will not rely on visuals to communicate if they have the ability to use spoken language.

The level of speech development varies by learner. Regrettably, some will never develop sufficient speech skills to become what we would consider competent speakers. Some will use a combination of visuals and spoken words or phrases. Some individuals make so much progress that they no longer need visuals to communicate. Regardless of the scope of their progress, we believe that visual language enables learners to reach their full potential for speech.

By now, readers should have a general idea of how the VEM, the VOM, and the VIM can be used to help learners with ASD. We go into greater detail on the practical aspects of applying these modes in Chapter 6. First, however, we describe how the VIP can be used as an assessment tool in Chapters 4 and 5.

Three Therapy Models

The complexity of the communication problems associated with the ASD population demand that instructors conceptualize therapeutic approaches to communication disorders in three ways. The *fix-it* model aims to correct the underlying source of the learner's disorder. The *compensation* model aims to give the learner alternative ways to handle the existing disorder. The *bypass* model circumvents the disorder with an alternative approach.

  The Visual Immersion Program may follow all three models, depending on the learner's developmental capabilities. It is important to continually assess the learner's response to intervention and modify the therapeutic approaches as appropriate.

  Fix-it model. For some individuals with ASD, the VIP serves as a remedial tool that strongly supports the development of receptive and expressive speech. Until the advent of augmentative communication approaches for learners with ASD this was the exclusive model of intervention Understandably, this is the outcome that all parents and instructors hope for.

  Compensation model. Most commonly, visuals serve to complement, support, and enhance the learner's ability to understand and speak in effect compensating for their communication deficits. In some cases, the continued supplementation offered by this approach may lead to comprehension and production that does not require accompanying visual supports. In fact, for some people, there is a steady and predictable improvement in communication.

  Bypass model. For individuals who are unable to develop the ability to speak, the VIP provides an alternative way to communicate, bypassing traditional speech in the same way sign language bypasses speech for a deaf person. The bypass model is an example of the purest form of augmentative communication.

  Regardless of which model the VIP most closely follows for a particular learner, instructors and parents should always bear in mind that the program's goal is to enable the learner to communicate and function as effectively as possible within his environment. It is understandable that many parents will hope for a complete fix, but they should be prepared if the therapy ultimately serves to compensate for the learner's speech difficulty or bypass it entirely. In every case the goal of intervention is to provide the individual with ASD the most appropriate and richest communication system available to him.

References

Bondy, A. S., & Frost, L. (1994). The Picture Exchange Communication System. *Focus on Autistic Behavior, 9*, 1–9.

Bondy, A. S., & Frost, L. A. (1998). The Picture Exchange Communication System. *Seminars in Speech and Language, 19*, 373–398.

Charlop-Christy, M., Carpenter, M., Le, L., LeBlanc, L., & Kellet, K. (2002). Using the Picture Exchange Communication System (PECS) with children with autism: Assessment of PECS acquisition, speech, social-communicative behavior, and problem behavior. *Journal of Applied Behavioral Analysis, 35*(3), 213–231.

Dexter, M. (1998). *The effect of storybook aided language stimulation on the communicative output of children with PDD-NOS.* Unpublished doctoral dissertation, Johns Hopkins University, Baltimore.

Fitzgerald, E. (1949). *Straight language for the deaf.* Washington, DC: The Volta Review.

Frost, L., & Bondy, A. S. (1994). *PECS: The Picture Exchange Communication System training manual.* Cherry Hill, NJ: Pyramid Educational Consultants.

Goldberg, H. R., & Fenton, J. (Eds.). (n.d.). *Aphonic communication for those with cerebral palsy.* New York: United Cerebral Palsy Association.

Goossens, C., Crain, S. S., & Elder, P. S. (1992). *Engineering the preschool environment for interactive, symbolic communication.* Birmingham, AL: Southeast Augmentative Communication Conference Publications.

Light, J., Drager, K., McCarthy, J., Mellott, S., Parrish, C., Parsons, A., et al. (2004). Performance of typically developing four and five year old children with AAC systems using different language organization techniques. *Augmentative and Alternative Communication, 20*, 63–88.

Luria, A. R. (1980). *Higher cortical functions in man.* New York: Basic Books.

MacDuff, G. S., Krantz, P. J., & McClanahan, L. E. (1993). Teaching children with autism to use photographic activity schedules: Maintenance and generalization of complex behavior chains. *Journal of Applied Behavior Analysis. 26*, 89–97.

McDonald, E., & Schultz, A. (1973). Communication boards for cerebral palsied children. *Journal of Speech and Hearing Disorders, 38*, 73–88.

Mirenda, P., & Erikson, K. A., (2000). Augmentative communication and literacy. In A. M. Wetherby & B. M. Prizant (Eds.), *Autistic spectrum disorders: A transactional developmental perspective* (pp. 333–367). Baltimore: Paul H. Brookes.

Pierce, K., & Schriebman, L. (1994) Teaching daily living skills to children with autism in unsupervised settings through pictorial management. *Journal of Applied Behavioral Analysis, 27*, 471–482.

Quill, K. A. (1995). Visually cued instruction for children with autism and pervasive developmental disorders. *Focus on Autistic Behavior, 10*(3), 10–20.

Romski, M., & Sevcik, R. (1996). *Breaking the speech barrier: Language development through augmented means.* Baltimore: Paul H. Brookes.

Schuler, A., & Baldwin, M. (1981). Nonspeech communication and childhood autism. *Language, Speech and Hearing Services in the Schools, 12*, 246–257.

Shane, H. C. (2006). Using visual scene displays to improve communication and communication instruction in persons with Autism Spectrum Disorders. *Perspectives in Augmentative and Alternative Communication, 15*(1), 8–13.

Shane, H. C., Douglas M. L. (2002, November). *Investigation into the use of intelligent agents in children evidencing autism.* Presentation at the annual meeting of the American Speech-Language-Hearing Association; Chicago, IL.

Vicker, B. (1974). *Nonoral communication system project: 1964/1973.* Iowa City: Campus Stores, Publishers, University of Iowa.

Wood, L., Lasker, J., Siegel-Causey, E., Beukelman, D., & Ball, L. (1998). An input framework for augmentative communication. *Augmentative and Alternative Communication, 14,* 261–267.

4

Assessment

Part 1: Visual Skills and Other Key Skills

Individuals with ASD are a challenging population to assess, especially those with severe developmental disabilities. A lack of linguistic competence may make it hard for them to understand a task or question's meaning or to formulate and communicate a response. They also often struggle with the fundamentals of testing procedures—the need to sit at a table, follow directions, answer questions, do one's best, and so on. In some cases, the difficulty they have as "test takers" masks existing linguistic competence. Whether the obstacles are primarily due to language or test-taking problems, clinicians and teachers are often stymied by how to best collect baseline data for this population.

Although we recognize the obstacles, we believe it is possible to systematically assess learners with ASD, and that doing so is critical for successful treatment. After all, without an awareness of a learner's abilities, it is impossible to know which areas therapy should focus on, choose the appropriate level of spoken language and communication support during instruction, and recognize whether a learner is making progress. Simply put, assessment drives instruction.

In this chapter, we review the methods we use to evaluate learners with ASD. Not surprisingly, we place a strong emphasis on visual skills, because we believe they are critical to improving communication. Although the tests we focus on are typically carried out by speech and language pathologists, the information may be relevant for anyone who works with individuals with ASD, including teachers, teacher's assistants, psychologists, and parents. For simplicity's sake, we refer to anyone who assesses a learner's skills as an evaluator.

Obstacles to Assessment

A number of factors can impede the differential assessment of communication difficulties experienced by individuals with ASD, including lack of speech, executive function difficulties, anxiety about unfamiliar people and situations, and skill scatter.

Lack of Speech

Spoken expression is typically used as a window into communication competence, and is a common means for evaluating an individual's language skills. Typically, diagnostic approaches rely on verbal communication to gain insight into both speech competence and language capability, beginning with tests that determine if spoken language is understood and at what level. These tests expect a behavioral response (usually verbal or gestural) to some spoken instruction, which assumes the learner understands and can act on the commands associated with a test protocol such as "point to," "show me," or "repeat." However, the fact that more than half of learners with ASD are nonspeaking means that speech output often is not available as a diagnostic tool. Common diagnostic tests that cannot be done because of restricted speech output include:

Auditory processing tests. Many tests that evaluate auditory processing skills require learners to speak to indicate whether they are able to take in auditory stimuli, draw conclusions, and respond appropriately.

Verbal cloze tests. A cloze test is a comprehension and expression exercise involving stimuli with certain words deleted and needing to be replaced. Diagnostic tests often use a spoken cloze test to see how well the learner can integrate semantic and syntactic understanding to complete verbally presented information.

Language sample tests. Representative samples of the learner's utterances are often used to analyze and evaluate developmental language levels and deficits areas.

One-word expressive language tests. Many assessments include diagnostic tasks that rely on the learner to give a spoken response to an array of stimuli.

Sentence repetition tests. Several diagnostic procedures use sentence repetition to evaluate the learner's understanding of semantic and syntactic language. The inability of some individuals with ASD to speak eliminates this option. At the same time, some learners who do not generate speech on their own are able to repeat long strings of words (echoic behavior). Although typically developing children are unlikely to be able to repeat a sentence that has semantic relationships and a grammatical form that exceeds their syntactic level of understanding, individuals with autism who display echoic behavior can repeat long strings of phonological information outside their understanding of the semantic and syntactic elements contained within the sentence.

Tests for apraxia of speech. Even though apraxia of speech is often suggested as the explanation for speechlessness in individuals with autism, that differential assessment can only be based on specific spoken error patterns, and those patterns can only be analyzed when a person actually speaks. A definitive diagnosis of apraxia of speech depends largely on an adequate speech sample. Furthermore, the very foundation of an apraxia of speech assessment (Darley, Aronson, & Brown, 1975; Duffy, 2005 depends on a cooperative participant who repeats a specific and detailed battery of speech sounds, phrases, and sentences. We believe apraxia of speech is an overdiagnosed phenomenon.

Apraxia of Speech: An Overdiagnosed Disorder

In recent years, a large number of learners with significant speech difficulties have received a diagnosis known as developmental apraxia of speech. In our view, individuals with autism are often incorrectly diagnosed with this condition, which can lead to misguided treatment that squanders opportunities for genuine improvement in communication skills. Following is a brief explanation intended to help instructors recognize apraxia of speech and distinguish it from autism.

Apraxia of speech is a neurological disorder characterized by the inability to program accurately the successive movements necessary for motor speech production. It is a motor planning disorder and not related to muscle strength, range, or coordination. The disorder can coexist with autism or occur independently.

Potential signs of apraxia of speech may be evident in infancy, such as difficulties sucking and swallowing and problems transitioning from liquid to solid food. Infants later correctly diagnosed with developmental apraxia of speech often were "silent babies" who did not babble or cry. Once they get older, children with apraxia of speech often have very specific speech difficulties, including the following:

- They may be unable to make particular speech sounds, such as fricatives (*th, v,* or *h*), affricates (such as the *ch*-sounds in church and the *j*-sound in joy), and sibilants (*s, sh, z,* or *zh*).
- They may have trouble with words of increasing length; if an instructor says the word "zip" and asks the learner to repeat it, he may be able to do so, but may falter when asked to repeat "zipper" or "zippering."
- They often repeat errors inconsistently, pronouncing a word correctly at one attempt and mispronouncing it on the next.
- They often can be seen groping for a particular word and struggling to produce it.
- They often have "islands of fluency," such as the ability to count, list the days of the week, and produce certain phrases without difficulty.

We believe learners who have difficulty speaking are often diagnosed with apraxia of speech because it appears to explain their speech problems. It is likely the trend toward overdiagnosing this condition for individuals with autism stems in part from the popularity of Facilitated Communication in the 1990s. At the time, "apraxia" was often offered as the reason individuals could not independently point to letters (or speak). This misconception was then generalized from limb apraxia to apraxia of speech.

The diagnosis of apraxia of speech is often given prematurely, before a child has had sufficient opportunity to learn to speak and before he exhibits enough symptoms for an evaluator to make a reasoned diagnosis. Toddlers who lag slightly behind their peers in speech development, for example, may be given a diagnosis of apraxia of speech. One year later, however, they may show significant improvement in their speech production.

More commonly, we see the diagnosis of apraxia of speech given along with the diagnosis of autism. In such cases, the child's speech difficulties can be attributed to the fact that individuals with ASD often start speaking later than typically developing children. As their speech emerges the unusual articulation and prosody patterns they produce are generally the result of a lack of practice and not praxis. As a result, they miss many early speech milestones, which makes their speech awkward when they do start talking. With therapy, learners with ASD can improve their speech performance and learn to articulate more clearly.

The following chart highlights key ways in which apraxia of speech differs from autism.

Key Differences Between Apraxia of Speech and Autism	
Apraxia of Speech	**Autism**
Speech programming problem	Language processing problem
Make speech errors inconsistently	Usually make the same speech errors repeatedly (i.e., errors patterns are consistent)
Individuals not usually echolalic	Individuals often echolalic
Speech progresses slowly with therapy, often plateauing after slight gains	Speech improvement follows a steady course
May have additional motor planning problems	Don't necessarily have motor skills problems

Executive Function Difficulties

Executive function refers to a set of meta-cognitive processes that allow an individual to adapt his behaviors to meet challenges and accomplish goals, by deciding what activities to attend to and choosing strategies to complete goal-oriented tasks. Executive function enables a person to plan and organize activities, direct his attention, and persist to complete a task, as well as to inhibit distractions and monitor thoughts to work more effectively. Learners with ASD often have poor executive skills and cannot adapt their behavior to successfully address a task's demands.

Executive skills include seven areas: attention, working memory, inhibition of competing stimuli (distractibility), task implementation, performance monitoring, task shifting, and automaticity. Although the evaluator may not formally address executive skills, it is helpful to be aware of these skills during assessment.

Anxiety About Unfamiliar People and Situations

Individuals with ASD are often anxious when confronted with new situations and unfamiliar people. The prospect of testing may prompt or exacerbate obsessive compulsive behavior (OCB); self-stimulatory behaviors (rocking, spinning, hand slapping, etc.); perseverative behaviors (repeating a behavior when it is no longer appropriate, such as remaining focused on a prior task or repeating words, etc.); and escape behaviors (running away, having a temper tantrum to get a time out, etc.). Such behaviors are less likely to occur if the learner is familiar with the evaluator and the assessment routine, so whenever possible assessment should be done by an individual who the learner already is familiar with through either a visual schedule or a personal meeting.

Skill Scatter

The wide disparity often found in a learner's skills, a phenomenon known as "skill scatter," is another factor contributing to assessment challenges. Although most children, including those with speech and language deficits, tend to follow a predictable pattern of development (even if it is delayed), learners with ASD often display a surprising and unpredictable range of skill acquisition. For example, a 3-year-old may have the decoding skills of a 7-year-old when reading and the comprehension skills of an 18-month-old.

Testing Strategies and Key Assessment Principles

Exploring communication competence generally involves using one or more testing strategies. The three most common behavioral testing techniques used by speech and language pathologists are interviews, observational checklists, and diagnostic protocols.

Interviews. Interviews in the context of assessment are attempts to gather information from a third party familiar with the learner, such as parents and teachers. For an interview to generate useful information, it is essential that historical and observational information be as accurate as possible. Biased reporting or information distorted by emotion will be misleading and may interfere with a well-informed diagnostic picture. The more specific and objective questions are, the less likely this is to occur.

Observational checklists. Observational checklists document the learner's skills and behaviors in a specific domain or environment. They do not, however, include information regarding performance quality.

Diagnostic protocols. This refers to a range of tests selected to evaluate specific aspects of the learner's communication skills. For such tests to be effective the evaluator may need to modify them. It is critical that the evaluator be completely familiar with the administration, scoring, and interpretation of the materials. When deviating from recommended procedures or introducing self-made materials or materials compiled from multiple sources, the evaluator should have specific reasons for doing so and know how to interpret the learner's reaction to modified procedures and materials. The evaluator also needs to be able to sort out when a learner's failure to relate to or perform a task is a function of not understanding a task's requirements or its level of complexity.

Three Assessment Principles

Three key principles underlie our approach to assessment:

1. Standardized Tests Are Ideal, But Adapted Tests Are Still Valuable

Standardized tests use uniform procedures for administration and scoring to ensure that the results from different evaluators are comparable. Often they are either norm-referenced or criterion-referenced. Norm-referenced tests (NRTs) are designed to highlight achievement or developmental differences between learners to provide a reliable estimate of how a learner performs in comparison to same-age peers. Criterion-referenced tests (CRTs), by contrast, report how well learners are doing relative to a predetermined performance level on a specified set of educational goals or outcomes.

Standardized tests should be used when the learner is able to understand the task and the requirements for responding to a stimulus item and has the cognitive and language ability to effectively participate in the standardized testing protocol. In sum, the student needs to demonstrate these four executive skills:

- task recognition
- procedural knowledge of testing situation
- inhibition of excessive off-task behavior
- ability to sustain attention to task.

Due to the difficulties learners with ASD often have in following directions and maintaining attention, in many cases standardized testing simply is not possible, and it is necessary to adopt a more informal approach and modify tests in ways that invalidate the testing method. Examples include testing in shorter intervals, using materials the learner is familiar with instead of those that come with the test, introducing visual supports, and presenting questions in multiple ways.

These modifications also invalidate percentile ranks, making it harder to compare an individual's progress with peers. Information gathered from adapted tests is nonetheless helpful in establishing a baseline, determining an approximation of developmental levels, and evaluating an individual's progress over time. The evaluator should always bear in mind that the goal is to get an inventory of the learner's language skills in various contexts, not to measure how well he can take a test.

Knowing how well a learner can sit at a table and participate in an activity such as test taking is not irrelevant. However, in this context it is more important to learn about language competence than test taking skills. An evaluator may observe, for example, that a learner demonstrates a particular skill while playing in the waiting room (such as organizing toys or responding to his name), but fares poorly when seated at a table for testing. In such cases, the evaluator should indicate that the learner is capable of the skill but also note the conditions under which he can and cannot do it.

When standardized scoring is invalidated, it is helpful to access an alternative response measurement system that is sensitive to the unique set of learning behaviors of individuals with ASD, such as the Performance Accuracy and Independence Response System (PAIRS).

2. Assessment Should Be Ongoing

Any evaluation should be considered a snapshot of the learner's abilities on that day, bearing in mind that if the learner is tested when he is having a bad day or is uncooperative, the results may not reflect his true skills. As noted earlier, regular assessment is needed to have benchmarks to measure an individual's progress. We believe that *every* treatment session should include an assessment component, and that instructors should make daily notes on the progress of every individual they work with. Once a learner has demonstrated mastery of a

---

The Performance Accuracy and Independence Response System

The Performance Accuracy and Independence Response System (PAIRS) is an innovative diagnostic tool that is highly sensitive to the particular profile of learning behaviors associated with individuals with ASD (Kearns et al., 2005). Specifically, PAIRS attempts to measure how well and independently individuals function in educational and clinical contexts given their level of functioning, so that appropriate adjustments can be made in the learning environment.

PAIRS focuses on how well a learner performs educational activities and how much support she or he receives from a teacher or staff member. To measure these aspects of learning, the tool uses two rating scales: a seven-point scale of accuracy and independence of responding (AI Scale) and a five-point participation rating scale (P Code). For example, the evaluator lists the type of assists the learner needs to perform a task, such as through a nonsymbolic reenactment of a physical hand-over-hand assist, or through a symbolic, conventional gesture such as pointing.

certain skill, therapy can move forward to more advanced skills.

3. No Single Assessment Currently Exists for Evaluating Learners with ASD

Assessment of the communication skills of learners with ASD continues to evolve; to date, there is no single diagnostic protocol that evaluates all domains in speech, language, and visual representational understanding, or even a consensus on which tests should be conducted. For now, evaluators must rely on existing tests, adapting them for the specific population they interact with. To help instructors develop an effective battery of tests, where appropriate we have included the names of some of the existing tests we find useful.

Assessment for Placement in Visual Immersion Program

A range of diagnostic information is needed for the appropriate placement of a learner into the Visual Immersion Program. In this chapter, we describe methods for collecting information in six areas: general history, spoken language, visual language, visual representation, reading, and observational learning. We have included a VIP Assessment Protocol Checklist at the end of this chapter that may be helpful in completing an assessment (Appendix 4A).

1. General History

The evaluator questions the learner's parents about the following:

- medical history (including past and current medications)
- developmental history (including motor acquisition, language development, any loss of language or skills, eating difficulties, and toileting)
- educational history (including early intervention, preschool, present school placement, current services and type of programming [e.g., Floortime, ABA, etc.])
- social history (including relevant information on parents, siblings, caregivers, pets, and participation in social or sports clubs)
- preferred and nonpreferred foods, toys, and activities
- manner of communication (use of gestures, visual symbols, text, and speech)
- pragmatic purposes of communication (requesting, protesting, and commenting).

2. Spoken Language Assessment

The evaluator should assess the learner's spoken language skills in terms of both comprehension (input/reception) and speech (output/expression). The focus is on determining whether the learner understands the various parts of speech and other key aspects of language. A number of standardized tests are available to test these skills, including the Preschool Language Scale (Zimmerman et al., 2002) and the CELF-4 (Wiig, Secord, & Semel, 1993, 2003).

If the learner is unable to participate in a formal assessment, the evaluator should be prepared to perform a nonstandardized assessment. The Monarch Natural Language Assessment, an observational checklist that evaluates receptive and expressive skills needed to manage functional communication, provides an example of a nonstandardized assessment (Appendix A).

During the assessment, the evaluator should keep well-documented information on delays in the learner's response time to auditory information (known as processing time latency). This information can be collected while presenting tasks that involve a simple direction, such as "put the ball in the box" or "give Mommy a kiss." The evaluator notes how many seconds elapse before the learner carries out the request. Some individuals with ASD show lengthy delays in response time—5 or 10 seconds is not uncommon, and we have encountered delays up to 20 seconds—so it is important not to misinterpret a lack of understanding before allowing enough time to process auditory input.

If there is a delay, the evaluator may want to repeat test stimuli using an auditory trainer that reduces ambient noise and creates a more positive figure/ground ratio. The evaluator notes whether using the device improves accuracy and/or cuts the response delay and by how much.

The evaluator should use developmental milestones as a reference for assessing the learner's acquisition of speech and language skills. For example, the learner may be able to answer "who" questions (a skill typically developing children master by age two-and-a-half), but not be able to answer a yes/no question (which typically developing children master by age two). This information, while highlighting the scatter in the learner's skills, also provides valuable information on acquired skills that can be shaped to enhance therapy. Appendix B (Chapman, 1981) lists the age at which typically developing children acquire the yes/no interrogative and "wh" questions.

3. Visual Language Assessment

The VIP is only an effective and appropriate intervention if the use of visual cues can lead to improved performance in the expressive, instruction, and organizational modes. To this end, the following series of initial questions relating to each area should be considered. An overall positive reaction to these inquiries suggests looking further into the use of a visual approach to communication and learning.

Visual Expressive Mode (VEM)

Speech Production
1. Is this individual's speech ineffective in most speaking situations?
2. Does this individual produce a limited amount of speech?
3. Is this individual's speech mostly unintelligible?
4. Does this individual self-limit speech production?
5. Does this individual speak or attempt to speak while pointing to photos, graphic symbols, or words?
6. If visual supports have been introduced, has this led the individual to produce more speech?

Communication Intent
1. Does this individual seem frustrated because he or she is unable to get his or her needs met?
2. Is this individual aware that intentionally pointing to, handing over, or indicating some representation is the means to acquire an item?
3. Does this individual bring you to the location of a desired item or activity?

Behavior
1. Do you suspect that aggressive or self-injurious behaviors, if they occur, are related to difficulty with communication?

Visual Instruction Mode (VIM)

1. Does use of visual cues improve this individual's ability to recognize an object, a directive, or an activity?
2. Does use of visual supports improve this individual's ability to understand spoken language?
3. Does this individual require additional time to process spoken language?
4. Does this individual have a language comprehension and processing disorder?

Visual Organization Mode (VOM)

Schedules
1. Is this individual's understanding of a daily schedule aided by visual supports?
2. Does use of visual supports seem to reduce the surprise associated with changes in routine or transitions to new activities?

Independence
1. Can this individual use the visual supports to independently follow a daily schedule?

Sequenced Learning
1. Does use of visual supports improve this individual's ability to understand a sequenced activity?
2. Is this individual's understanding of a sequenced activity aided by visual supports?

Independence
1. Can this individual use identified visual supports to independently follow the sequenced activity?

4. Visual Representation Assessment

The essence of the visual representation assessment is to determine the learner's understanding of the relationship between concepts/information (generally conveyed through verbal speech) and a visual equivalent.

Differential assessment is a critical element of an effective evaluation. The VIP assessment requires careful consideration of the learner's ability to respond to information presented only through spoken language, contrasted with his performance with the addition of visual supports. As with all assessments, the evaluator determines the highest level of accuracy the learner is able to achieve when given the least amount of assistive support.

An effective assessment of visual representation skills should cover comprehension of:

■ directives with and without visuals
■ levels of representation
■ grammatical categories and concepts.

Directives With and Without Visuals

Evaluators should informally explore whether the learner's comprehension of concepts such as size, shape, color, and spatial relationships (i.e., prepositions) increases when visual supports are provided. For example, the evaluator can arrange plastic chips of various colors (e.g., red, blue, yellow, and green), shapes (squares and circles), and sizes (small and large) on a tabletop and ask the learner to point to or manipulate a particular chip (e.g., "touch the small red square chip" or "put the large green square next to the yellow circle").[1] In a subsequent trial, the evaluator repeats the request, this time while presenting a scene cue (e.g., a laminated strip containing a visual image of the correct response). The evaluator observes whether the addition of the scene cue improves the learner's accuracy and rate of responding.

If the visual supports do improve the results, the evaluator should next assess whether the learner is merely performing a one-to-one exact match of the chips to the scene cue or is differentiating and analyzing elements contained within the scene cue. To find out, the evaluator uses element cues that specify size, shape and color, as in the two examples below (Figure 4-1). Such cues require the learner to demonstrate understanding of the semantic relationship between the elements and apply this knowledge by selecting the correct corresponding chip.

Example 1. The evaluator shows the following strip and asks the learner to "point to the big circle" (Figure 4-1A).

Example 2. The evaluator shows the following strip and asks the learner to "point to the blue square" (Figure 4-1B).

---

[1]The Token Test for Children (DiSimoni, 1978) is a more formal way of structuring this task.

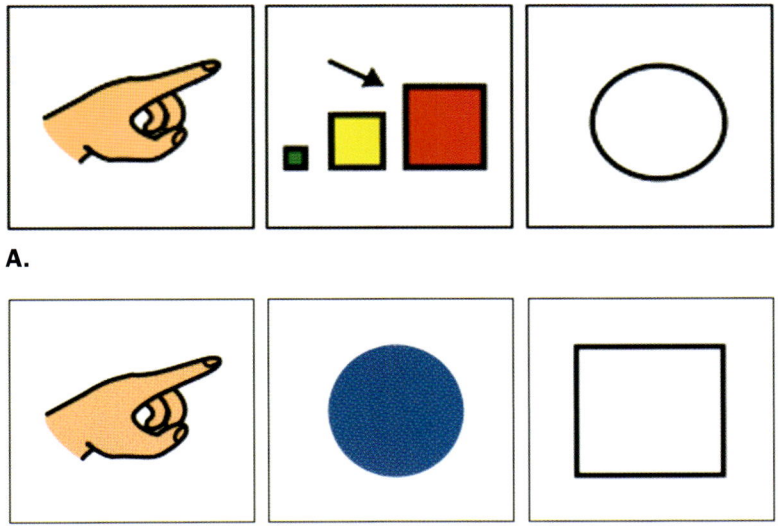

A.

B.

Figure 4–1. Examples of *Token Test* (DiSimoni, 1988) modification using visual symbols denoting size and shape: **A.** Point to the big circle). **B.** Point to the blue square. (From The Picture Communication Symbols ©1981–2007 by Mayer-Johnson LLC. All Rights Reserved Worldwide. Used with permission.)

Levels of Representation

A learner shows understanding of visual relationships by identifying a visual representation equivalent to a sample the evaluator presents. Sorting and matching exercises are an effective way for a learner to point out the equivalency of one level of representation to another and organize items having stimulus equivalence into similar storage bins. There are five levels of sorting; for all five the evaluator begins by placing three objects in separate bins in a horizontal array in front of the learner. The objects should be relatively uninteresting and easily "sortable"; we use a collection of skeleton keys, plastic knives, and small rubber horse figures.

Level 1: Learner matches identical stimuli (objects/proxy). The evaluator hands the learner three objects that are exact matches to the objects in the bins and directs him to place the objects in the appropriate bins. "Direct" can mean either a spoken command or, if necessary, a spoken command combined with a gesture or hands-on physical assistance demonstrating how to sort the items. (Here and in general, the evaluator should begin with minimal assistance and gradually add more help as needed because the goal of the assessment is to determine the highest level at which a learner can accomplish a task.)

Level 2: Learner matches 3D representation to object. The evaluator hands the learner 3D representations of the objects in the bins and directs him to place the 3D representations in the appropriate bins. (3D representations are described in Chapter 2.)

Level 3: Learner matches photograph to object. The evaluator hands the learner photographs of the objects in the bins and directs him to place the photographs in the appropriate bins.

Level 4: Learner matches colored picture to object. The evaluator hands the learner colored drawings of the objects in the bins and directs him to place the colored drawings in the appropriate bins.

Level 5: Learner matches line drawing to object. The evaluator hands the learner line drawings of the objects in the bins and directs him to place the line drawings in the appropriate bin.

Grammatical Categories and Concepts

Sorting routines can help determine the learner's understanding of levels of representation associated with nouns that are primarily objects. It is also important to know the level of representation for other noun themes (people and places) as well as other grammatical categories. To determine the most appropriate types of visual representations to use, evaluators must consider the learner's understanding of the relationship of a visual equivalent to a number of different grammatical categories and concepts. For each of the following grammatical categories, we cover four practical areas: materials needed, levels of representation, type of representation, and assessment procedures.

Nouns. The issue here is mainly one of knowing the appropriate level of representation—can the object, person, or place be represented by a photo, a line drawing, an animated cartoon, and so forth?

Materials:
- For tabletop setting: figurines and objects
- For virtual setting: multimedia video clips and animated software
- For natural environment: designated people, objects, and places

Level of representation: Set of element cues that portray each of the people, objects, and/or places from each of the above settings.

Type of representation: Static (nonmoving) scene cues.

Assessment procedures: A learner can demonstrate understanding of nouns through a number of effective strategies including matching (symbol to object, object to symbol, symbol to symbol); physically retrieving an item portrayed by a visual cue; looking toward or pointing to a person when a visual cue is provided; and moving to location represented by the visual cue (particularly important if a visual cue is being used to signify a transition).

Verbs. Verb understanding can be assessed through scene cues that portray an actor acting on an object, for example, the boy is climbing the ladder, or the girl is pushing the wagon.

Materials:
- For tabletop setting: figurines and objects
- For virtual setting: multimedia video clips and animated software
- For natural environment: designated people, objects, and places.

Level of representation: Set of visual action cues that portray each of the action concepts depicted from each of the above settings.

Type of representation: Static and dynamic (moving) scene cues (e.g., animation showing pulling, pushing, etc.). The evaluator needs to carefully collect data on the learner's response to the type of representation. Some learners need the highest degree of representation (animation showing pulling, pushing, etc.), whereas other learners can interpret dynamic action from a still photograph.

Assessment procedures: Generally within a static or dynamic image, a figurine is engaged in movement (jumping) or acting on an object (pulling a wagon, placing an object in a vessel). The learner is expected, in response to a static or dynamic cue, to imitate the activity portrayed by the character. There are three levels:

Level 1: Matching to static scene cues. The evaluator tests the learner's ability to recognize elements within the scenes by asking him to match items (such as ladder to ladder and truck to truck). Scene cues are initially evaluated at a static level by asking the learner to use the objects on the table to re-enact particular actions ("show me the boy lying on the bed"). Lying on the bed is a static action, and the learner can reproduce this by copying exactly what he sees in the picture.

Level 2: Matching to dynamic scene cues. The evaluator tests the learner's ability to recognize scene cues at a dynamic level by asking him to recreate the action with figures ("show me the boy pushing the cup"). To successfully demonstrate understanding of the action of "pushing," the learner needs to interpret the concept and intent of the dynamic movement of "pushing" even though it was represented in a static photograph.

Level 3: Matching to animated-dynamic scene cues. We have found it helpful to produce dynamic scene cues that show arecognizable character (such as Kermit the Frog or Woody from "Toy Story") doing activities such as climbing a ladder and pulling a wagon. Such dynamic scenes can be created through short video vignettes that are transferred to a computer. When possible, it is preferable to use a digital video camera, which allows you to isolate a scene cue to serve as a static representation of the animation.

First, the evaluator makes the same objects that will appear in the animation available to the learner (a Kermit figurine, a toy ladder, a wagon, etc.), and places them on a table between the learner and the computer screen. Then the evaluator makes a series of verbal requests intended to see if the learner can identify and manipulate these objects, such as "point to the ladder," "show me Kermit climbing the ladder," "put Kermit on the wagon," "show me the big white bowl," and "make him jump." Next, the evaluator shows the dynamic scenes on the computer screen and repeats these requests, observing whether showing the scene improves the learner's ability to respond to the verbal requests.

While doing this test, the evaluator also collects information on whether the learner is able to attend to the screen, shift his gaze from the screen to the objects in front of him, as well as reproduce the behavior he has witnessed.

The evaluator also evaluates the quality of the learner's imitation by observing whether he is imitating the behavior shown in the scene cue with or without understanding its meaning and intent. For example, when the learner is asked to "show me Kermit climbing the ladder," if he correctly places Kermit on the ladder but does not move the toy up the ladder, he is just imitating the behavior without understanding its meaning. If he correctly places Kermit and also makes him move up the ladder, he understands the meaning and intention of the scene cue.

The evaluator also should assess whether scene cues are effective in environments other than the tabletop. Directives given in familiar contexts should be avoided. Instead, give directives that ask the learner to use common objects in uncommon ways. For example, ask him to "put your shoes in the bathtub" or "throw the paper under the table." Then compare his performance when a scene cue depicting shoes in a bathtub and paper under the table is provided.

Prepositions. Prepositions can be assessed with the use of scene cues similar to those used to assess action verbs. The scene is constructed to specify a spatial relationship between the actor and an object, for example, the girl is sitting *on* the chair, or the book is *under* the table. The evaluator assesses prepositional understanding with scene cues at all three levels described above.

Adjectives. Level 1 and Level 3 scene cues lend themselves well to assessing understanding of adjectives. The scenes are constructed to contain contrasting descriptors that correspond to objects for the learner to select. For example, the learner matches either a small, blue truck or a large, blue truck to the corresponding scene cue to evaluate the ability to differentiate the descriptor of size. Similarly, the scene could contrast color (e.g., a large red truck contrasted with a large blue truck) to differentiate the learner's response to descriptors of color.

5. Reading

The learner's reading skills should be assessed in nine areas: concepts of print, phonological awareness, logo recognition, decoding skill, semantic understanding, automaticity, fluency, and sentence and text comprehension. Existing reading tests that may helpful include the Oral Written Language Scales (OWLS) (Carrow-Woolfolk, 1995), the Woodcock Reading Mastery Tests-Revised (WRMT-R; Woodcock, 1987), the Comprehensive Test of Auditory Phonological Processing (CTOPP) (Wagner et al., 1999), and the Phonological Awareness Test (PAT) (Robertson et al., 1997).

Concepts of Print

Concepts of print is the awareness of print and its functions, such as left-to-right directionality and the understanding that print carries a message and that words are made up of letters. To assess this skill, the evaluator sits next to the learner at a table with a book that has one or two sentences per page and clear illustrations or pictures corresponding to the text. The evaluator begins by handing the book to the learner upside down or sideways and observing if he corrects the orientation. Next, the evaluator reads the story's first page while pointing at the corresponding pictures, noting if the learner's gaze moves from the print to the picture. Finally, the evaluator gestures for the learner to turn the page, observing whether he acts on the gesture and turns a single page or indiscriminately flips the pages.

Phonological Awareness

Phonological awareness is the ability to recognize and manipulate the sound structure of language. It involves familiarity with a range of issues related to the sounds of words and word parts, including identifying and manipulating parts of spoken language (such as words, syllables, and sounds). This includes rhyming; identifying the first, middle, and final sounds in words; and the ability to blend constituent sounds into words. Phonological awareness skills are the foundation for typical acquisition of decoding skills for reading.

Standardized assessments such as the Comprehensive Test of Phonological Processing (CTOPP) and the Phonological Awareness Test (PAT) can be used to formally assess phonological awareness skills. If the learner is unable to participate in a formal assessment, the evaluator can informally assess these same skills. For example, the evaluator can assess word awareness by telling the learner a specific word and asking him to clap when he hears that word in a sentence. Rhyming skills can be evaluated receptively by asking him if he thinks two words rhyme (e.g., "Does *train* rhyme with *rain*?") and expressively by asking the learner to generate a rhyme (e.g., "Tell me a word that rhymes with *cat*").

Logo Recognition

Logo recognition is the ability to recognize that a logo stands for a known item. The evaluator shows the learner several familiar logos and asks him to point to a specific logo. Many learners with ASD easily recognize a familiar logo and demonstrate understanding that the logo stands for a preferred item. This ability can be shaped into forming broader symbol understanding.

Decoding Skill

Decoding is the ability to map sounds (phonemes) to letters (graphemes) and then blend the constituent parts into a word. The learner may be able to apply his knowledge of spelling (orthographic) patterns to the word and map sounds to the pattern, but still may not be referencing the meaning associated with the word. To assess decoding skill the evaluator shows the learner words he is unlikely to be familiar with, but that follow standard pronunciation rules (such as "mite," "propane," and "extemporize"), and asks him to read them aloud.

Reading with Meaning

Some learners with ASD can decode well but lack the ability to comprehend text. In other words, they read without meaning. To begin assessing reading for meaning, the evaluator first shows the learner a series of printed words he is likely to be familiar with by sight (such as his name, "mom," and "book") and asks the learner to read them aloud. The evaluator then asks the learner to match the word to the appropriate object or picture (from a display of numerous objects or pictures). If the learner recognizes the configuration of the word and maps sounds to it but cannot match it to the appropriate object or picture, then he has not demonstrated an ability to read with meaning.

Automaticity

Automaticity is reading with accuracy and speed. The evaluator observes how quickly and accurately the learner reads a series of words and phrases. Automaticity is an important step in enabling a learner to move from focusing his attention on decoding words to understanding their meaning.

Fluency

Fluency is moving beyond automaticity to reading effortlessly. It includes appropriate prosody (melody, rate, and intonation) and the appropriate chunking of phrases, which leads to an ability to anticipate what may come next. The evaluator assesses whether the learner reads sentences as if he understands them, based on his phrasing and overall continuity. A robotic reading style is often a sign of poor fluency, whereas varying one's tone of voice and pausing at appropriate places between phrases and sentences indicates an understanding of the material being read. These fluency skills help the learner construct meaning and intent from written passages.

Sentence and Text Comprehension

Reading is ultimately about comprehension. It is important to assess how well the learner is able to use text as a method for receiving meaningful information. To assess comprehension the learner reads a short passage describing a scene or activity, and the evaluator asks questions intended to determine if he understood the passage. The evaluator can start with simple questions that quote directly from the passage but leave off the final word. If the learner is successful with this activity, the evaluator asks more open-ended questions, such as who, what, where, when, why, and how.

For students who have reading skills but are not able to be tested on a standardized assessment, a reading skills checklist can be used (Figure 4–2).

Concepts of print

☐ Yes
☐ No

> Is the learner interested in books?

☐ Yes
☐ No

> Does the learner hold a book with the correct orientation?

☐ Yes
☐ No

> Does the learner look at the pages?

Comments:

☐ Yes
☐ No

> Does the learner look at the pictures in the book?

☐ Yes
☐ No

> Does the learner attend to the book when being read to?

Comments:

Figure 4–2. Reading Skills Checklist *(continues)*

Phonological Awareness:

☐ Yes
☐ No
Is the learner aware of words in sentences?

☐ Yes
☐ No
Is the learner aware of syllables in words?

☐ Yes
☐ No
Is the learner aware of sounds in words?

☐ Yes
☐ No
Can the learner identify rhyming words?

☐ Yes
☐ No
Can the learner generate rhyming words?

☐ Yes
☐ No
Can the learner identify the first sound in a word?

☐ Yes
☐ No
Can the learner identify the last sound in a word?

☐ Yes
☐ No
Can the learner blend sounds to reconstruct a word?

Comments:

Figure 4–2. *continued*

6. Observational Learning

Observational learning refers to the learner's ability to absorb new information from watching others. The evaluator assesses how well the learner can imitate behavior and also looks at whether different instructional methods affect his performance. There are four areas to look at: imitation as a surface copying behavior, role-reversal imitation, instructional delivery preference, and electronic screen media (ESM) skills.

Imitation as a Surface Copying Behavior

The evaluator acts out simple actions, such as waving arms or tossing a ball in a box, and asks the learner to do the same thing he or she is doing.

Role-Reversal Imitation

The goal here is to determine if the learner understands a task's intent or is merely copying the other person. The evaluator can do this by making a minor mistake after asking the learner to imitate what he or she is doing. For example, the evaluator might explain through a gesture or a verbal directive, "We need to put all the red pens in this box." The evaluator puts several red pens in the box and watches to see if the learner does the same. Then the evaluator accidentally places the next pen outside the box. If the learner copies this mistake, he shows he does not understand the task's intent. If he corrects the error by continuing to place his pens in the box, then it is likely that he does understand the task.

Instructional Delivery Preference

The evaluator should experiment to determine in which type of learning scenarios the learner seems to do best. For example, it is helpful to compare the learner's performance when he receives direct instruction from a "live" person versus when he receives the identical instruction from a person on a videotape. Many individuals with ASD fare better with videotaped instruction.

Electronic Screen Media (ESM) Evaluation

The evaluation of observational skills should also include a review of the learner's familiarity with electronic screen media, such as television, movies, and computers. This information, which a parent can provide, may help determine which information delivery systems the learner is most likely to benefit from. The ESM Questionnaire (Table 4–1) elicits this information and can help the mentor decide on the type of media that may be of instructional value.

In the next chapter, we look at how an evaluator can assess learners' experiential skills.

Table 4–1. Electronic Media Interest Questionnaire

Television	Movies
Does your child watch television at home? Yes/No If yes, please complete questions listed below:	Does your child watch movies? Yes/No If yes, please complete questions listed below:
Please list titles of your child's favorite television programs:	Please list titles of your child's favorite movies:

My child: (Please check all that apply)
- ☐ Repeats/attempts to repeat words from a television program/movie
- ☐ Sings/hums songs from preferred television program/movie
- ☐ Imitates movements on program/movie
- ☐ Tunes out distractions (e.g., name being called) while watching program/movie
- ☐ Re-enacts events on the screen with stuffed animals, toys, or figures
- ☐ Focuses more on remote control or buttons on television rather than the program/movie
- ☐ Focuses on written language on television screen more than other features
- ☐ Responds to emotional events and/or facial expressions in program/movie
- ☐ Views select shows/movies repeatedly, to the exclusion of other shows/activities

How are movies/television programs used in your home? (Check all that apply)
- ☐ An educational tool for the child
- ☐ A means of occupying the child so you can complete a task
- ☐ Recreation
- ☐ A reward
- ☐ Other (please describe):

Computer

School	*Home*
Does your child use a computer at school? Yes/No	Do you have a working computer your child uses at home? Yes/No
How frequently does your child use the computer at school?	How frequently does your child use the computer at home?
Purpose(s) of computer use: (Check all that apply) ☐ Educational tool ☐ Reward ☐ Communication (e.g., computer-based voice output device, specialized software)	Purpose(s) of computer use: (Check all that apply) ☐ Educational tool ☐ Reward ☐ Communication (e.g., computer-based voice output device, specialized software)

Table 4–1. *continued*

Please list your child's preferred software programs:

How does your child access the computer? (Check all that apply)
☐ Mouse   ☐ Keyboard
☐ Adaptive access (e.g., IntelliKeys,   ☐ My child does not independently
touch window, etc.)   access the computer

References

Carrow-Woolfolk, E. (1995). *Oral Written Language Scales (OWLS).* Circle Pines, MN: American Guidance Service.

Chapman, R. S. (1981). Children's answers to wh questions. In J. Miller (Ed.), *Assessing language comprehension in children: Experimental procedures.* Baltimore: University Park Press.

Darley, F., Aronson, A., & Brown, J. (1975). *Motor speech disorders.* Philadelphia: W. B. Saunders.

DiSimoni, F. (1978). *The Token Test for Children.* Austin, TX: Pro-Ed.

Duffy, J. R. (2005). *Motor speech disorders: Substrates, differential diagnosis, and management* (2nd ed.). St. Louis, MO: Mosby.

Kearns K., Shane, H. C., Weiss-Kapp, S., & Tourian M. (2005, November). *Managing autism outcomes: The participation, accuracy, and independence scales.* Presentation at the annual meeting of the American Speech-Language-Hearing Association; Philadelphia.

Robertson, C., & Salter, W. (1997) The Phonological Awareness Test (PAT). East Moline, IL: Lingui Systems.

Wagner R. K., Torgesen, J. K., & Rashotte, Carol A. (1999). The Comprehensive Test of Auditory Phonological Processing (CTOPP). Austin, TX: Pro-Ed.

Wiig, E., Secord, W., & Semel, E. (1993). *Clinical Evaluation of Language Function-Pre-School.* San Antonio, TX: The Psychological Corporation.

Wiig, E., Secord, W., & Semel, E. (2003) *Clinical Evaluation of Language Function-4 (CELF-4).* San Antonio, TX: The Psychological Corporation.

Woodcock, R. (1987). *The Woodcock Reading Mastery Tests-Revised (WRMT).* Circle Pines, MN: American Guidance Service.

Zimmerman, I. L., Steiner, V. G., & Pond, R. E. (2002). *Pre-School Language Scale-4* (4th ed.). San Antonio, TX: The Psychological Corporation.

APPENDIX 4A

VIP Assessment Protocol Checklist

The following checklist can be used during or after an assessment, to ensure that all areas are covered.

1. General History　　　　　　　　　　　　　_____

2. Spoken Language Assessment　　　　　　　_____

3. Visual Language Assessment　　　　　　　　_____

4. Visual Representation Assessment　　　　　_____

   A. Directives with and without visual supports　_____

   B. Levels of representation　　　　　　　　_____

   C. Grammatical categories and concepts　　_____

5. Reading Assessment　　　　　　　　　　　_____

   A. Concepts of print　　　　　　　　　　_____

   B. Phonological awareness　　　　　　　　_____

   C. Logo recognition　　　　　　　　　　_____

   D. Decoding　　　　　　　　　　　　　_____

   E. Semantic understanding　　　　　　　_____

   F. Automaticity　　　　　　　　　　　　_____

   G. Fluency　　　　　　　　　　　　　　_____

   H. Sentence and text comprehension　　　_____

6. Observational Learning Assessment　　　　_____

   A. Imitation as a copying behavior　　　　_____

   B. Role-reversal imitation　　　　　　　　_____

   C. Instructional delivery preference　　　　_____

   D. Electronic Screen Media questionnaire　_____

5

Assessment

Part 2: Experiential Knowledge

Despite limited language comprehension and expression skills, learners with ASD can often handle routine daily tasks (such as getting dressed, using a DVD player, drawing pictures, helping parents with chores, etc.) with relative ease, and in some cases better than typically developing children who are the same age. This ability to master how things work results from experiential knowledge—familiarity with the natural environment gained through experience and observation of ongoing occurrences.

Experiential knowledge can play a critical role in learners with ASD's language development, for this important reason: learners can gain experiential knowledge without the need for (nor do they necessarily benefit from) language, but once learned, experiential knowledge can be used to build language skills. To understand why this is the case, we need to look at both parts of this equation.

Learners with ASD Typically Gain Experiential Knowledge Without Benefit of Language

Experiential skills are inherently visual and physical in nature and therefore do not depend on the spoken language system to develop. Instead, individuals learn them through observation, experimentation (trial and error), as well as adult-directed instruction.

Consider, for example, how a child learns to negotiate his environment. As he encounters objects and people, he does not need to refer to their labels (nouns), nor does he need to know the names of actions (verbs) to act them out. For example, when he sees a door he does not consciously or unconsciously say to himself, "Hey, that is called a door. It is made of wood, and the metal items on the edges are called hinges." He just appreciates that because of his past observations and experiences with doors, he can pass through it or open and close it.

Similarly, a child learns to do more complex tasks, such as turning a light on and off and using a faucet to wash his hands, through observation and experimentation, without knowing the names of the elements involved. There is, in essence, a nonverbal relationship between the learner and the relevant objects (the light switch, the faucet, soap, etc.) that exists without any need for linguistic interpretation. Increasingly complex tasks that require steps in a sequence, such as shoe tying or bicycle riding, do typically require some language instruction, but observation and experimentation nonetheless play a major role.

A critical element of experiential skills is that they are almost always goal-oriented, so the result serves as a built-in reward that motivates the learner to master the task (the lights come on, water comes out the faucet, shoes can now be worn, etc.). Learners with ASD can be single-minded in pursuing mastery of a task, often to the exclusion of other demands on their attention and are therefore more willing than typically developing children to accept temporary failure as they learn new routines. As a result, they often develop a wide repertoire of experiential skills—they know where household items are kept, use latches and doorways, can open the window to allow air in, help themselves to food in refrigerators and cabinets, know to bring a chair over and stand on it to reach something on a high shelf, can navigate a computer mouse, and so forth. The ability to perform such skills is often referred to as procedural or schema knowledge (Kamhi, 1991).

Once Learned, Experiential Knowledge Can Be Used to Build Language Skills

Although experiential knowledge can be sufficient to accomplish a task, symbolic knowledge is needed when an individual wants to tell others about what he sees, feels, or thinks. The actual expression or output of symbolic knowledge is what we refer to as the Visual Expression Mode (VEM). Experiential knowledge provides a strong basis for such expression because it is much easier for a learner to apply language to a concept he already has experience with—and thus some level of understanding of—than to a concept he has not experienced and does not understand.

Consider the verb "open." Depending on the context, open can mean pull (opening the refrigerator), push (opening a swinging door), or rip and tear (opening a bag of chips). Attempts to teach the word "open" to an individual who is unable to perform these tasks is likely to be a confusing and fruitless exercise. However, a learner who can already do all three tasks is likely to learn the word more easily because he knows that the concept of openness is always associated with confronting some type of barrier.

The combination of the learner's familiarity with these experiences and an appropriate scene cue—such as an animated character opening a door while saying "I'm opening the door" or an action element cue (symbol representing "open") presented during the course of opening—is an effective way to map a symbolic representation to the concept of "open." This principle of experiential knowledge preceding language growth can also be applied to teaching all parts of speech.

Although there is a general awareness that learners with ASD often have strong experiential knowledge, instructors have made little effort to capitalize on this phenomenon. We believe it is vital to systematically identify and assess experiential knowledge, so that symbolic language can be mapped onto it and instruction can focus on improving skills a learner has yet to master.

In this chapter, we show how to assess experiential knowledge, using a questionnaire we developed called the Experiential Knowledge Profile (EKP). Before presenting the EKP, we briefly examine some research that supports making experiential knowledge a key component of therapy for learners with ASD.

development depends on a cultural context that structures events for a child and a child's capacity to learn from this cultural structuring (Vygotsky, 1962). In terms of learners with ASD, the developmental pragmatics movement of the 1970s and 1980s emphasized that the social context of naturally occurring routines was critical to language development (Bates, 1976, 1979). In the 1990s, Applied Behavioral Analysis (ABA) theorists—after initially taking the view that individuals with ASD could not easily learn in natural environments because of learning and attention problems—developed the "natural language paradigm," which highlighted the effectiveness of learning from routines that recur in everyday life with family and peers (Schreibman & Pierce, 1993).

Previous Research

Although experiential skills are not currently a major focus of autism treatment, existing research on learners with and without ASD provides a basis for their relevance. Important points in this research include the following:

Context Is Critical to Language Development

A number of researchers have highlighted the important role of context in language development—that is, the potential advantages of the real or "natural" environments over tabletop or classroom environments. In the 1930s, the pioneering developmental psychologist Lev Vygotsky observed that language

Children Learn by Observation

In the famous "Bobo Doll" experiment by Albert Bandura, nearly 90% of children who witnessed an adult hitting a doll later imitated the adult's behavior, without any instruction or reward (Bandura & Walters, 1963). An important follow-up study found that children were as likely to imitate the adult's behavior when they watched it on film. Although Bandura's studies are often used to cite television and film's negative influence on children, the studies also demonstrate that young learners quickly pick up tasks by observation and that media can be an effective teaching tool.

Our own research confirms learners with ASD's interest in observational learning through electronic screen media, or ESM[1] (Shane & Albert, 2005).

---

[1]Observational learning through electronic screen media by learners with ASD may also be referred to as video modeling.

Our survey found that individuals with ASD often:

- spend more time with media (television, movies, computers, video games, etc.) than other activities
- demonstrate strong experiential skills
- prefer animated characters to humans
- and imitate words and sounds they hear on ESM

Parents' comments often highlight their children's strong interest in media. We frequently hear observations such as "If I could put myself inside a TV, he'd listen to me" and "If Winnie the Pooh told my daughter to do something, she'd do it."

Individuals with ASD Often Learn Better When They Lead

Developmental pragmatics views the learner as an active participant who directs his own learning rather than someone led by a teacher with a specific reinforcement schedule. Similarly, the central feature of the popular ASD therapy Floortime is for the instructor to follow the learner's lead. Floortime recognizes that unlike typically developing individuals, learners with ASD often do not recognize that adults' statements and actions are intentional and important and, as a result, do not follow an instructor's lead (Greenspan & Wieder, 1998).

The Experiential Knowledge Profile

The EKP, which is filled out by a learner's parents, caregivers, and teachers, evaluates three aspects of experiential abilities.

1. Experiential Knowledge in Specific Environments

The assessment identifies skills the learner has mastered in five environments: the kitchen, bathroom, bedroom, living room, and classroom. For example, in the kitchen, can he do tasks such as washing hands, drinking, eating, and simple food preparation? In the classroom, can he do tasks such as sitting down, writing, and listening quietly to the teacher?

For each skill, the parent or teacher indicates whether it was learned through observation (learner-acquired) or instruction (adult-directed). It is not necessarily a negative if the individual learned a task through instruction, as it shows he is able to interpret the instructor's intent by re-enacting a task and applying it in a meaningful way.

2. Assistance Needed

The assessment identifies the skills the learner needs help with and what type of assistance is typically provided. There are five types of assists: physical (hand-over-hand guided direction) which is presymbolic and symbolic based assists including: gestural (pointing, indicating, pantomime); visual (photographs, line drawings, etc.); verbal (spoken language); and written (text). If the learner is capable of doing a task without such assistance but needs encouragement to motivate him to initiate the task, there is a "needs reminder" option.

3. Concept Awareness Across Multiple Environments

The assessment identifies which general concepts the learner uses in more than one environment. Examples include arriving, eating, opening, closing, and replacing items.

Completing the EKP

The EKP is included in Appendix C. Using the following instructions, parents and caregivers fill out the form addressing EKP routines that occur within the home, and teachers and staff fill out the form addressing EKP routines that occur at school.

Step 1. Review the functions in the Routine column and determine which functions the learner can perform.

Step 2. Decide whether the skill was Learner-Acquired, Adult-Directed, or N/A. Use the Learner-Acquired column for skills the individual learned primarily on his or her own, with no instruction from you. Use the Adult-Directed column if the child required a lot of direction from you as he or she learned that skill. Check N/A if the child has not been introduced to or has not acquired the skill.

Step 3. In either the Learner-Acquired or Adult-Directed section, check off whether the child has "mastered" the skill or mastery is "in progress." (If you have chosen N/A for a particular skill, skip this step and step 4 for that skill.)

Step 4. For all functions the learner has not mastered, indicate in the appropriate "prompted" column which type of assistance he or she needs. (Such functions are usually Adult Directed but can be Learner Acquired in cases in which learners use a trial and error method to acquire a skill independently, but

benefit from an assist to initiate or produce a step in the routine.) Use the appropriate letter code from the following list of the five prompt types:

P for Physical Assist: A physical assist requires hand-over-hand guided direction in assisting the child in initiating the task.

G for Gestural Assist: A gestural assist uses conventional gestures such as pointing, indicating, or pantomime to assist the child in initiating a task.

Vs for Visual Assist: A visual assist uses visual supports such as photographs or line drawings to assist the child in initiating a task.

Vr for Verbal Assist: A verbal assist uses spoken language to assist the child in initiating a task.

Wr for Written Assist: A written assist uses text to assist the child in initiating a task.

Example. If you are in the process of teaching the learner to open the refrigerator and he or she requires you to point to the refrigerator to help him or her do so, that line in the EKP would be filled out as in Table 5-1.

Scoring the Results

The Function portion is scored by circling the corresponding line item numbers on the Profile onto the following **Function Key** (Table 5-2).

Step 1. Circle **in red** the corresponding number and letter of the functions within the routines that were checked off in the Learner-Acquired column.

Table 5–1. Example of EKP Used to Teach Opening the Refrigerator Door

	Beverage Routine	Learner-Acquired Skills				Adult-Directed Skills			
		Mastered	In Progress	Prompted	N/A	Mastered	In Progress	Prompted	N/A
B-1	**Open** *the refrigerator door*					X	G		

Table 5–2. Function Key

	Kitchen	Bathroom	Bedroom	Living Room	Classroom
Move	A-1, A-2	A-3, A-4, A-5, A-6, A-7			A-8, A-9, A-10, A-11
Put	E-1, E-2, E-3	E-4	E-5		E-6, E-7, E-9, E-10, E-11
Transfer	F-1, F-2, F-3, F-4	F-5, F-6			F-7
Consume	G-1				G-2, G-3
Insert	H-1	H-2		H-3	H-4, H-5, H-6
Determine	I-1			I-2, I-3	
Mix	J-1	J-2			
Position	L-1, L-2, L-3, L-4, L-5	L-6, L-7, L-8, L-9			L-10, L-11, L-12, L-13
Wipe	0-1, 0-2,	0-3, 0-4, 0-5			
Personal Care		P-1, P-2, P-3			
Undress		Q-1, Q-2	Q-3, Q-4		Q-5, Q-6, Q-7, Q-8, Q-9
Dress		R-1, R-2	R-3, R-4, R-5		
Play		S-1			
Attend					T-1
Work					U-1
Greet					V-1, V-2
Part					W-1

Step 2. Circle **in blue** the corresponding number and letter of the functions within the routines that were checked off in the Adult-Directed column.

Step 3. Count up the total number of both Learner-Acquired and Adult-Directed columns and record the total number in the corresponding boxes in the **Summary Function Key** (Table 5-3).

Step 4. Count the number and type of assists in the Learner Acquired column and enter the total of each type of assist into the **Learner Acquired Assist Key** (Table 5-4).

Step 5. Count the number and type of assists in the Adult Directed column and enter the total of each type of assist into the **Adult Directed Assist Key** (Table 5-5).

Step 6. Enter the completed number of Routines into the **Completed Routines Key** (Tables 5-6, 5-7, 5-8, 5-9, and 5-10). Routines are considered completed if the Learner performs a minimum of 3 steps ending with the last step in the routine.

Applying the Results of the EKP to Plan Therapy

Information from the **EKP** combined with information from the VIP assessment is the basis for developing goals and objectives for visual language development at the appropriate level of symbolic representation for the learner.

Functions

The **Summary Function Key** provides the instructor with information regarding

Table 5–3. Summary Function Key

Number of Learner-Acquired Functions: ____	Number of Adult-Directed Functions: ____
Learner-acquired functions, which are circled in red, were learned independently	*Adult-directed functions, which are circled in blue, were learned by explicit adult direction*

Table 5–4. Learner-Acquired Assist Key

Assist for Learner-Acquired Functions	
These assists are used to retrieve or prompt an acquired function.	spoken: ____
	gestural: ____
	graphic: ____
	written: ____

Table 5–5. Adult Directed Assist Key

Assist for Adult-Directed Functions	
These assists are used to instruct while the Learner is acquiring the function	spoken:
	gestural:
	graphic:
	written:
	physical:

Table 5–6. Completed Routines Key for Kitchen Routines

	Complete
Beverage	
Snack	
Washing Hands	
Sitting at Kitchen Table	

Table 5–7. Completed Routines Key for Bathroom Routines

	Complete
Washing Hands	
Brushing Teeth	
Toileting	
Bathtub	

Table 5–8. Completed Routines Key for Bedroom Routines

	Complete
Putting Away Toys	
Dressing for the Day	
Undressing	
Dressing for Bed	

Table 5–9. Completed Routines Key for Living Room Routines

	Complete
Using a TV	
Using a VCR	
Using a Computer	

Table 5–10. Completed Routines for Classroom Routines

	Complete
Snacking: Drinking from a Juice Box	
Snacking: Eating from a Snack Bag	

the learner's repertoire of functional concepts. The key provides a visual summary of the learner's most well-established concept understanding of functions across multiple environments as well as identifying which functional concepts are not yet known or applied by him.

The functional concepts that are well-known and practiced by the learner are the ones onto which symbols, either spoken or visual can be mapped. The functional concepts that are not yet learned become the targets for developing conceptual understanding. Chapter 6 provides detailed information for designing therapy based on visual language and concept development goals identified through the EKP.

Nouns

Nouns for vocabulary building are chosen for their relevance to the function and environment in which the functions are being taught. For example, "refrigerator, glass, juice," and "table" may be selected as vocabulary items when teaching the function of "pour." The **EKP** provides a vocabulary list of noun items that are relevant to the functions contained within the assessment.

Prepositions

Each function in the **EKP** inventory has several prepositional interactions embedded into the performance of the function. Chapter 6 discusses the use of dynamic scene cues to teach prepositional concepts within the structure of performing the routine.

Prompts

The types of prompts needed by the learner to perform the functions in the **EKP** informs the instructor regarding which are the most effective assists for the learner in acquiring new information. This also identifies if the learner is still working at a presymbolic level and needs physical direction to complete a function, or if he is responsive to symbolic assists of gestural, visual, verbal, or written information. This information is used to identify appropriate scaffolds, cues and prompts before implementing therapy.

Sequencing Steps in a Routine

The learner's ability to perform a goal-oriented sequence when performing a routine informs the instructor of his skills in selective attention, allocation of attention to a task, ability to maintain a task, inhibition of competing stimuli, and monitoring of performance. It also provides a window into whether the learner can appreciate the benefit of his own actions. These skills reflect the learner's executive strategies and give evidence of his ability to adapt his behavior to effectively engage in learning.

Three Levels of Learners

Results from the questionnaire place learners into one of three levels:

Level I

Level I learners show no evidence of procedural understanding and cannot perform any experiential skills without physical assistance from an adult.

All experiential skills and procedural concepts need to be explicitly taught. Behaviors associated with Level I learners include the following:

- May not show awareness of his environment or other people
- May not understand relevance of procedures and routines to himself (i.e., seeing another person drink a glass of water does not prompt him to seek a drink for himself)
- May not be able to imitate another person's behavior
- May not understand task requirements (i.e., that getting a drink of water requires finding a cup, turning on the faucet, and filling the cup).

Level II

Level II learners have a range of experiential skills, most of which they gained through instruction (adult-acquired). They can perform some goal-oriented routines, but often require assistance. The type of assistance needed is usually symbolic, such as gestures and spoken and written language. Behaviors associated with Level II learners include the following:

- May have difficulty paying attention
- May be reluctant to initiate tasks
- May fail to complete routines, for several reasons (does not remember the end goal of a task; cannot plan steps needed to complete a sequence; does not understand the concepts of beginning, middle, and end because of problems with temporal processing)
- May have difficulty with symbolic representation, such as understanding the connection between a photo of a duck and an actual duck
- May have difficulty with relational aspects of language such as prepositions and adjectives.

Level III

Level III learners have a range of experiential skills, most of which they learned through observation (child-acquired). They use these skills in multiple environments. They are able to carry out complete goal-oriented routines, but may need an adult's gestural, visual, or spoken prompt to initiate the sequence. Behaviors associated with Level III learners include the following:

- May have difficulty paying attention
- May have difficulty recognizing a task's situational relevance
- May have difficulty perceiving similarity of established routines in novel settings (for example, a learner who can get a drink of water at home may get confused at a relative's house)
- May have difficulty with symbolic representation
- May have difficulty with relational aspects of language.

The intervention plan is tailored to the learner's level, with symbolic language mapped onto experiential knowledge. As we describe in detail in Chapter 6, intervention for Level I learners focuses on building basic vocabulary (nouns) through presymbolic re-enactments and teaching them to perform specific steps within a larger routine. Intervention for Level II learners uses visual symbols to build intermediate vocabulary (primarily

---

Parents' Perspective on the EKP

Parents often find the results of the Experiential Knowledge Profile encouraging. Results of conventional assessments of language and comprehension skills are often disappointing, as parents are frequently told their children have severe intellectual impairments (e.g., a 6-year-old with the language skills of a 3-year-old, or a 4-year-old with the fine motor skills of a 18-month-old). Such results may be especially upsetting in cases where parents see their children doing well at everyday tasks and routines. The EKP provides a measurable way of indicating that a child really has learned more than conventional evaluations show.

nouns, plus some other parts of speech) and teach entire routines once learners master specific steps within larger routines. Intervention for Level III learners uses visual symbols to build complex vocabulary (emphasizing verbs, prepositions, and adjectives) and teach the learner to initiate and carry out goal-oriented sequences. Regardless of the learner's level, the goal of intervention is for the learner to gain new skills that enable him to migrate to the next level.

References

Bandura, A., & Walters, R. H. (1963). *Social learning and personality development.* New York: Holt, Rinehart & Winston.

Bates, E. (1976). *Language and context: The acquisition of pragmatics.* San Diego, CA: Academic Press.

Bates, E. (1979). *The emergence of symbols: Cognition and communication in infancy.* San Diego, CA: Academic Press.

Greenspan, S. I., & Wieder, S. (1998). *The child with special needs: Encouraging intellectual and emotional growth.* Reading, MA: Addison Wesley Longman.

Kamhi, A. G. (1991) Causes and consequences of reading disability. In A. G Kamhi & H. W. Catts (Eds.), *Reading disabilities: A developmental perspective.* Needham Heights, MA: Allyn & Bacon.

Shane, H. C., & Albert, P. (2005, November). *Electronic screen media for persons with Autism Spectrum Disorders.* Presentation at the annual meeting of the American Speech-Language-Hearing Association; Philadelphia.

Schreibman, L., & Pierce, K. (1993). Achieving greater generalization of treatment effects in children with autism: Pivotal response training and self-management. *The Clinical Psychologist, 46,* 184–191.

Vygotsky, L. S. (1962). F. Hanfmann & G. Valar, Trans. *Thought and language.* Cambridge, MA: MIT Press.

6

Intervention

Applying the Three Modes of the VIP

In this chapter we discuss how instructors[1] can use the Visual Immersion Program to work with learners with autism. Intervention includes three routine-based language components designed to enhance communication:

- language instruction mapped to functional and relevant routines
- language expansion activities progressing through gestalt (whole) forms to analytically, based activities
- use of temporal displays to organize and anticipate activities and transitions.

Before covering these three components, we discuss some basic intervention principles and strategies, beginning with general guidelines for instructional objectives and areas of communication skill development.

General Instructional Objectives

1. **Every individual with ASD should learn to protest, refuse, and request effectively.** These three communication skills are essential to day-to-day function, and the ability to effectively

---

[1]As noted in Chapter 1, we use the term "instructor" to encompass all individuals who work with learners with autism, including teachers, teacher's assistants, occupational therapists, speech pathologists, psychologists, and parents. Exercises in this chapter carried out at home are most commonly taught by parents.

communicate them can help reduce problem behaviors.

We should point out that direct intervention is generally not needed for a person to communicate protests/refusals, or requests. Most everyone has an innate ability to express these pragmatic functions without a formal language system. For example, an individual can protest or refuse by throwing objects, screaming, crying, running away, and so forth, and he can request by pulling someone to the location of the desired item or standing beside it.

However, the introduction of a symbol allows for greater specificity without the need for interpretation. The instructor's role is to interpret and identify these meaningful behaviors and then help the learner express them through symbols. Ideally, the individual will learn to protest, refuse, and request with speech or visual symbols, but, if this is not possible, at minimum he can learn to communicate physically through gestures. If possible, everyone the learner encounters will be able to understand his protests, refusals, and requests, but it is essential that the specifics of such nonverbal communications, at the very least, be clear to those familiar with him.

The foundation for many communication programs is the pragmatic function of requesting. Such programs are generally successful because instructors know what is important to a learner through observation (i.e., they observe which objects he prefers to interact with or the food he prefers to eat) and then introduce symbols to reflect those same preferred items.

2. **Every individual should learn to respond to basic directives**

(such as stop, no, point, sit, come, show me, etc.). The learner's ability to respond to basic directives (expressed through spoken or visual language) helps with further learning, and improves behavioral management. In addition, understanding and responding to language such as "stop" and "no" plays a critical safety role.

3. **Every individual who works with a learner with ASD should learn to interpret when he is happy, sad, and interested.** The communication of basic emotions is an important part of the daily life of the learner. Interpreting these basic emotions helps guide the instructor on how to best interact with the learner and can help the instructor ward off behavioral outbursts. For example, if the learner is upset, it may be a good time to work on simple exercises to calm him down and if he is happy it may be a good time to return to work or begin work on new or more challenging tasks. Because learners with ASD often have difficulty commenting on their emotions, the instructor's ability to interpret the learner's affective state is critical here. It is not unusual for the expression of affect to initially come about through effective interpretation, with the instructor then building the use of symbolic expression on this innate foundation

4. **Every individual should have the opportunity to make smooth transitions from one activity to another.** To feel calm and organized people need to be

able to anticipate their next encounter. Visual supports enable learners with ASD to understand, anticipate and envision what is going to happen next, which helps them adapt better to their schedule and surroundings and reduces problem behaviors.

Two additional objectives may not always be achievable but instructors should strive to attain them.

5. **Individuals should learn to comment, describe, ask questions, and engage in conversation.**
   These pragmatic communication skills provide substance for conversation and insight into what the learner sees, hears, and believes. To engage in them, the learner needs to appreciate that his communication partner is an "intentional being," that is, an individual with his own perspective. Many learners with ASD have an inherent difficulty understanding the perspective of others, making these pragmatic skills more difficult to attain.

Learners with basic conversational skills are more likely to develop more complex communication skills and pragmatic abilities.

6. **Individuals should learn basic social conventions such as greetings and partings.**
   Greetings and partings are social conventions that signal awareness of another's presence and the understanding that others desire acknowledgment. To appreciate this, the learner needs to recognize other people's perspectives and also

pick up on social cues (such as a person opening a door, putting on or taking off her coat, etc.). The learner also needs to be able to interpret environmental signals that suggest the appropriate greeting or parting (such as knowing when to hug, shake hands, or nod to other people).

It is important here to distinguish between imitation and actual understanding of social concepts. For example, individuals with ASD are often directed to "say goodbye," "say hello," or "say thank you" during social encounters. However, simply echoing such a request from others, while a simulation of social conventions, does not mean the learner appreciates the social conventions that underlie their use.

Areas of Communication Skill Development

We find it helpful to conceptualize intervention as addressing three general areas of the learner's communication skills: basic skills (Type 1), language concepts and skills (Type 2), and pragmatic skills (Type 3).

Basic Communication Skills (Type 1)

A portion of therapy should be dedicated to helping the learner improve his ability to communicate basic needs and emotions as they arise, such as his physical needs (hunger, thirst, using the bathroom, that he is hurt), his emotional state (happy, sad, interested, angry, etc.), what he wants, where he wants to go, what he does and does not want to do, and so forth. In many cases, the learner communicates these needs without any effort, and it is just a matter of the instructor interpreting behavior, body language, facial expression, and utterances. For example, the learner may communicate thirst by standing in front of the refrigerator or that he is upset by screaming.

Many caregivers demonstrate impressive interpretive skills, gauging learners' emotional state and needs through sounds, movements, gestures, and affect. We view this interpreted behavior as having a great deal of communicative value, as it sets the stage for more advanced communication when nuances are disentangled by careful observation and thoughtful reflection. However, as noted earlier, intervention should aim to help the learner communicate at more advanced and socially acceptable levels (e.g., through gestures, use of visual symbols, and speech). The setting for improving Type 1 communication is usually within the natural environment. Specific suggestions for improving Type 1 communication are described in Chapter 7.

Language Concepts and Skills (Type 2)

Therapy focus is on helping the learner develop specific language skills, such as enlarging his vocabulary and improving his understanding of linguistic structure, concepts, and meaning. Improving these skills requires explicit instruction, with goals based on comprehensive assessments. The setting for improving Type 2 communication is usually the tabletop and/or the virtual environment.

Use and Generalization of Communication Skills (Type 3)

At times, intervention focuses on helping the learner improve his ability to interact with the natural environment through spontaneous use of already acquired gestures and spoken, visual, and written language (for greetings and partings, complex requests, comments, conversational exchanges, etc.). Improving such communication skills essentially means helping the learner take what he can do independently and elaborate and apply it meaningfully in appropriate situations. Type 3 skill development is related to what the psychologist Lev Vygotsky referred to as the "zone of proximal development"—the gap between a learner's current development level and his potential level of development when working with an instructor or more competent peer[2] (Vygotsky, 1962). The setting for Type 3 communication is usually the natural environment.

Instructors should work on all three areas of communication skill development depending on the needs of the learner. Most commonly, the instructor introduces new language skills and concepts (Type 2). Once they are stabilized, the instructor works with the learner to integrate them into essential (Type 1) and generalization (Type 3) skills.

---

[2]The formal definition of the zone of proximal development is the distance between the actual development level as determined by independent problem solving and the level of potential development as determined through problem solving under adult guidance, or in collaboration with more capable peers (Vyogotsky, 1978).

One common instructional error is overemphasizing Type 2 at the expense of Type 3. Some instructors identify a series of goals and then work with the learner in a tabletop or virtual environment, checking off mastery of new skills one by one. However, instructors may neglect to work on having the learner apply these new skills in a meaningful way in the natural environment. As a result, even though the learner appears to be learning new skills in the structured setting (the tabletop or the computer), his ability to communicate in other contexts (real-world situations) does not significantly improve. Most often, the problem results from the individual being a strong associative learner; he can reproduce what the instructor is doing in the specific situation where he learned it but does not understand the underlying meaning of what he learned.

Additional Intervention Principles and Guidelines

We now review some additional general intervention principles and guidelines. Note that much of this information applies to all therapy for individuals with ASD, not just the Visual Immersion Program.

Assessment Drives Instruction (Revisited)

As discussed in Chapter 4, without an awareness of a learner's abilities, it is impossible to know which areas therapy should focus on and recognize whether a learner is making progress. We reiterate this point because it not uncommon for instructors to begin therapy without assessing a learner's comprehension levels, or to take the time to do an assessment but then largely disregard the results and apply a one-size-fits-all approach. Instructors should always be aware of which skills the learner has already acquired and which skills he is likely to acquire next.

Treatment Should Be "Scaffolded" to Suit the Child

Scaffolds are assists specifically tailored to the individual's needs before therapy starts. To be effective, the instructor must be cognizant of the learner's speech and language capacity as well as which levels and types of visual representation the learner mastered, which contexts he uses them in, and decide what types of visual cues and supports are needed to get the most successful performance from the learner. This should flow naturally from the assessment results.

Proper scaffolding requires considerable planning on the instructor's part, but it is time well spent. Skipping this vital step increases the likelihood that therapy will be less effective, as the learner is likely to become bored if tasks are too easy and frustrated if they are too hard. Bear in mind that the window of opportunity for teaching learners with ASD is often small; once an individual becomes upset and throws a tantrum it is difficult to calm him down and resume instruction. One behavioral meltdown can torpedo an entire session or day's work.

As a practical matter, it is often advisable to begin each instructional session with an activity the learner has mastered that is just below a slightly more advanced skill he cannot yet do. This lays the framework for success because it gives the learner an opportunity to practice relevant skills he can do correctly before moving to a more complex skill. For example, if the learner has previously shown he can match photos to objects but has not yet matched line drawings to objects, then the instructor should spend some time having him matching photos to objects before introducing line drawings. This exercise revisits the same general skills the learner needs for the new task (i.e., sitting at a table and matching objects to appropriate symbolic representations).

Instruction Should Always Be Aimed at Moving the Learner Forward

Whatever the starting point, therapy should always be aimed at bringing the learner to the next level. This means moving the learner from gestalt processing toward increasing analytical processing (e.g., from understanding symbols in the context of whole scenes to understanding discrete element symbols), as well as toward increasingly natural environments (e.g., from the virtual and tabletop environments to the natural environment).

Begin with the Maximum Number of Assists Needed, and Then Work Toward the Minimum Number

In general, instructors should offer significant guidance when showing the learner a new task, including physical assistance when necessary. This type of support ensures the learner appreciates the proper way to perform the task. Once the learner can perform the task with physical assistance, the instructor can gradually ease off and encourage the learner to do the task more independently (a process known as fading).

This approach reduces the likelihood of the learner "practicing his errors," that is, learning to do the task incorrectly, and then having difficulty breaking from repeatedly making the same mistake. This is a particular risk for individuals with ASD, as they are apt to repeat routines the same way once they have done them a few times.

Consider an instructor who wants to work on the learner's ability to match objects to photographs. The instructor, for example, might place a pencil, a paper clip, and a key on the table along with matching photographs of these objects and direct (or expect) him to put the objects on top of the photos. Instead of doing so, the learner may pick up the key and put it in his mouth. Rather than repeat this exercise, with the same likely result, the instructor might consider taking a step back to work on demonstrating the task or providing physical guidance on how to place an object onto a matching photograph. Once the learner demonstrates mastery of this skill, the instructor can reintroduce the unassisted matching task.

Effective Intervention Integrates All Aspects of the VIP

Although certain environments and tools are especially effective for teaching particular concepts, it is important to recognize that, in practice, instructors integrate all aspects of the VIP into therapy. It is not uncommon, for example, for one session to include use of multiple instructional settings (virtual, tabletop, and natural), all types of cues—element cues and scene cues (dynamic and static), and multiple displays (grid displays, whole scene displays, and mixed displays)—with frequent switching back and forth among settings and display types. (Readers may wish to refer back to Chapter 3 for definitions of these and other terms used in the VIP.)

Create a Symbol-Rich Environment

Critical to the VIP's success is the creation of a "symbol-rich environment" at home and in school and, whenever possible, in other environments like the family car and the homes of friends and relatives. This refers to an environment in which visual symbols clarify spoken language, help with transitions, and facilitate learning. A symbol-rich environment encourages opportunities for both expressive (VEM) and receptive (VIM) communication. We discuss this further later in this chapter, in the section on language expansion.

Not Every Communication Is an Instructional Moment

At times, instructors and parents should just focus on addressing the learner's needs, not improving communication skills or managing behavior. Communication should be easy; sometimes a request for a cookie is just a request for a cookie, not the initial step in a recipe for expan-

sion to a sentence such as "I want a cookie please." Viewing every communication as a learning opportunity can inadvertently dissuade the learner from attempting to communicate because such pressure is too uncomfortable and he feels too much pressure, especially when he is often struggling. On a practical level, it is impossible for the instructor to always have the ideal visual supports available to make every moment a teaching opportunity.

Use Language the Learner Will Understand

Comprehension is the foundation of successful communication and language improvement, so instructors should always bear in mind the learner's comprehension level. Unless the learner has demonstrated comprehension of complex sentences, instructors should use short, uncomplicated sentence constructions. Too often, instructors use the same speaking style they use with colleagues and typically developing children and mistakenly assume the learner understands. From the learner's perspective, it is as if the instructor is speaking a foreign language.

For example, an instructor might say, "John, we're going to go to the playground now, but before we go out I'll need you to put on your coat." A child who has not mastered complex sentence construction with time elements will not comprehend this. Instead, the instructor should first say, "John, we're going to the playground now." Once the learner shows he has understood this information, the instructor can say, "John, get your coat." When the learner returns with the coat, the instructor can say, "John, put on your coat." Note that a conversation display or relevant scene cues that depicts these events with visuals can clarify this exchange as well (Figure 6–1).

Avoid Robotic Instructions

Another common pitfall is overcompensating for the learner's comprehension deficit by dropping words from a sentence, such as articles and pronouns, leading to a robotic, staccato speaking style. For example, the instructor may say, "Want drink now?" instead of "Would you like a drink now?" There is no evidence that this linguistic abbreviation actually benefits comprehension. In fact, intonation and prosody are a part of every language system, and natural speech plays an important role in sentence comprehension. Accordingly, instructors should use full sentences suitable for the learner's comprehension level.

Attend to the Learner's "Distractibility"

Learners with ASD are often easily distracted, so it is important to be aware of factors that interrupt his attention and engineer an environment that reduces visual and auditory distractions. For learners with obsessive compulsive disorder, it is useful to identify and remove items they are likely to focus on. If attention is a persistent problem, it may be helpful to modify the listening environment. Comprehension often improves when the learner uses noise cancellation headphones that reduce ambient noise and allow him to hear the evaluator's voice through the headphones.

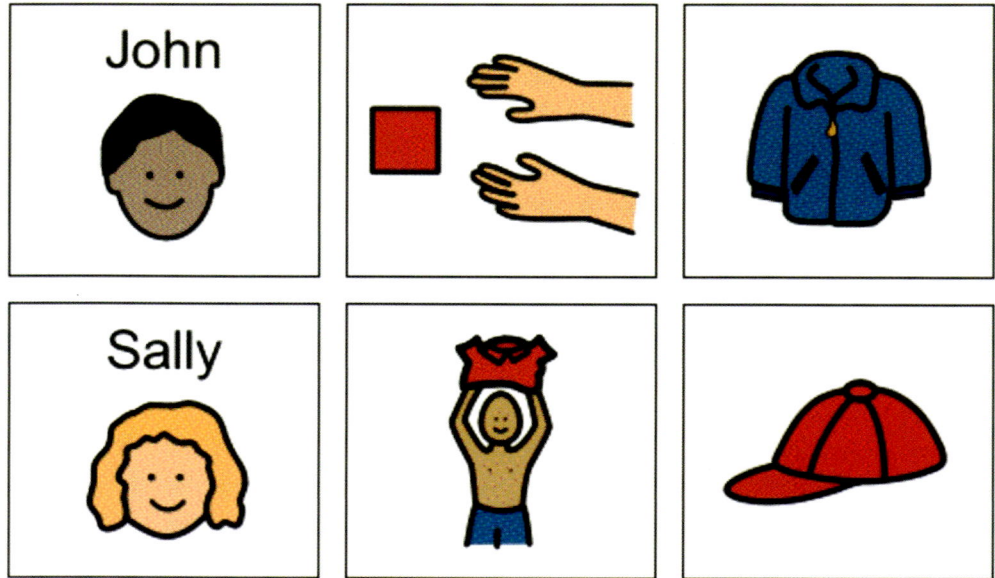

Figure 6–1. Example of a conversational display on the topic of preparation for recess. (From The Picture Communication Symbols ©1981–2007 by Mayer-Johnson LLC. All Rights Reserved Worldwide. Used with permission.)

Do Not Overstress Eye Contact

Although eye contact has important social value and for some learners is helpful in redirecting their attention to a task, instructors should not insist on it at all times. Not all learners need to make eye contact to pay attention and it is not always possible to equate eye contact with comprehension. As long as he is responding to the instructor's directives, there is no need to interrupt a lesson to demand that the learner "look at me now." Too often, instructors waste valuable time establishing eye contact that could be spent working on improving the learner's communication skills.

Teach Learners Four Key Hand Gestures

All individuals with ASD should have a way to indicate four essential concepts: *more* (recurrence), *help* (assistance), *stop* (termination), and *all done* (completion). One way to increase the likelihood that these concepts become part of a learner's learning repertoire is to use conventional American Sign Language gestures. These four gestures, which the learner's parents and instructors should also know and use, are critical for communicating basic needs and everyday functioning (although there is no need to introduce them if the learner can already express these four concepts with speech or visual representations).

To teach the gestures, instructors may need to physically shape the learner's hands and model the gestures. Instructors should not be concerned if the learner is unable to form his hands perfectly for each gesture. The important thing is that he is able to communicate these four concepts. When teaching the gesture for "more," make sure the learner understands that this gesture symbolizes recurrence; it should not be used to request new items.

Language Instruction Mapped to Routines

Intervention typically begins with work on the learner's ability to perform routines. This work accomplishes two broad objectives—the individual learns and practices new skills, and, equally important, he learns the language skills relevant to these routines, which ideally he can then generalize to other routines and other similar relevant experiences. For example, an individual who understands and can heed the directive "pour yourself a glass of water" may also be able to pour himself a glass of juice or pour his father a glass of water without specifically being shown how to do so.

The routines identified for instruction are selected based on the results of the Experiential Knowledge Profile (EKP) discussed in Chapter 5. Level 2 and Level 3 learners who are able to complete specific routines and the procedural functions contained within those routines are ready to begin mapping symbols to the procedural functions and objects within the routines. For example, if the learner is able to complete the routine of holding his toothbrush, squeezing the toothpaste onto the toothbrush, and brushing his teeth, this routine should be identified for instruction with the goal of mapping symbols to each element contained within the steps in the routine. Premade scene cues, mixed displays, and conversation displays are designed to emphasize the mapping of symbols to conceptual elements that are known to the learner such as the nouns ("bathroom, sink, toothbrush, toothpaste, towel"), verbs ("squeeze, brush, rinse, wipe"), and prepositions ("in, on, off").

EKP assessments that identify learners as Level 1 indicate their inability to complete routines or understand the meaning of procedural functions within routines. EKP results also may indicate that some Level 2 or Level 3 learners have not mastered the procedural functions within specific routines. In these instances, learners need to begin with instruction that supports concept development and understanding of the procedural elements within a specified routine.

The goal of routine-based instruction at this level is to give the learner multiple opportunities to observe the salient aspects of a goal-oriented routine and to supply multiple, highly scaffolded relevant opportunities to perform the routine. Initial instruction at this level should emphasize use of dynamic and premade scene cues for modeling while acting out the procedural steps within the goal-oriented routine. As the learner gains and stabilizes procedural understanding of the routine, as well as the functions of items used within the routine, he can begin learning to map symbol elements to the routine.

Language instruction for routines uses five types of visual tools: computer screen displays, premade scene cues, buildable scene cues and whole scene displays, mixed displays, and conversation displays. We begin our description of each instructional exercise with a listing of the exercise goal, the VIP mode (or modes) the exercise uses, and the materials needed. In general, if the learner cannot perform a particular step when directed to, the instructor should model the step for him or give him physical assists until he can perform it. In some cases, the instructor may need to go back to earlier steps in the exercise, switch to a less complex task, or switch to an earlier exercise.

Visual Immersion Program Instruction

The VIP is a multisensory structured visual language program that provides a comprehensive scope of visually based communication activities. Early activities are gestalt forms and assist the learner in gaining skills in both comprehension and expression of requests and comments through the use of dynamic and static scene cues. The learner progresses through carefully scaffolded activities with the goal of achieving independent and spontaneous use of element-based visuals for analytical processing and comprehension, as well as the use of elements for generating novel expressive constuctions for requesting and commenting within naturally occurring contexts.

Vocabulary expansion is systematic and is instructed for both comprehension and expression. It brings the learner through increasingly complex uses of vocabulary, beginning by identifying the appropriate levels of visual representation for the learner's vocabulary use. Subsequent goals include introducing multiple exemplars of specific vocabulary items and ultimately instructing in the relationship of vocabulary to the environmental contexts in which the items are likely to occur.

There are four basic principles to consider when implementing the VIP.

1. Routines for instruction should be selected for their relevance to the learner. In other words, the routines should include activities that provide him with multiple opportunities to practice his new skills in the context of the natural environment.

2. The learner's communication partner should consistently use the visuals to communicate with him not only during instruction, but conversationally throughout the natural context of the day. Similarly, the learner should be encouraged to use the visuals for requesting, commenting, and as a retrieval mechanism for performing multi-step goal-oriented, sequenced routines during the naturally occurring context of his day.

3. Once the learner has demonstrated proficiency using scene cues in performing a contextually based routine, the display containing the sequence of relevant scene cues should be placed in an area that is highly visible to the learner within the environment in which it occurs. For example, a scene display for making a sandwich can be placed on the counter where the materials are gathered and the sandwich is made.

4. Some learners will require a transitional activity, such as the matching tasks for levels of representation described later in the chapter, to assist them in appreciating the relationship between items they may have used in tabletop instruction and the items they are using in the natural environment. For example, the learner may need explicit instruction to understand that the toothbrush he is using in his bathroom at home has the same function as the one used when learning the routine in a tabletop activity at school.

Computer Screen Displays

The virtual environment (a computer screen) is often a good place to start working with learners with ASD, as they tend to have strong interest in computers (Shane & Alpert, 2005) and are less likely to be distracted by irrelevant information. Computer technology enables you to use a video clip to capture the salient aspects of a routine, break it into shorter segments, and create photos of screen shots of key moments in the routine.

Goal: To give the learner a structured opportunity to observe salient aspects of a routine (gestalt form).

Mode: Visual Instructional Mode (VIM)

Materials:
- computer loaded with the appropriate video clips and screen shots
- portable photo versions of screen shots
- actual objects used in routine.

Example: Opening a bag of chips.

Step 1: Begin by showing the learner a short video clip on the computer of a person performing the routine. This is an actual real-time depiction (i.e., a dynamic scene cue), which can be made with a digital video camera. For this example it might last 10 seconds, and include a woman picking up the bag, tearing it open, and pulling out a chip with her fingers. It may be necessary to replay the clip several times until you think the learner is attending to the routine.

Step 2: Determine the most relevant steps in the sequence using no more than three to five steps in the sequence. For example:

Segment 1: Woman picks up and holds bag of chips.

Segment 2: Woman tears the top off the bag of chips.

Segment 3: Woman pulls out one chip.

Step 3: Create screen shots that capture the essence of each segment (i.e., static scene cues). This would be a picture of the woman holding a bag of chips, a picture of the bag halfway open, and a picture of the woman pulling out one chip (Figure 6–2).

Step 4: Reconstruct the sequence by reenacting the routine for the learner (actually open a bag of chips on the table).

Step 5: Direct the learner to act out the sequence.

Note that it is important for these sequences of scene displays to be available for the learner to refer to in the environment in which they occur to assist him in generalization. Furthermore, the availability of the sequenced scene displays can be used to encourage the learner to independently initiate and complete the sequence. (This applies to the use of visual displays from every exercise.)

This exercise is effective for numerous simple routines, such as pouring a glass of water, putting an item in the garbage can, putting on gloves, and so on. In addition to video clips of actual people performing the routine, and depending on the learner's preference for animated characters, animated video clips can also be used.

Note that not all learners are interested in video monitors or computer screens, and computer screens and monitors are not always available for instruction. Also, some individuals learn tasks more effectively starting on the tabletop and then moving into the virtual environment. In some circumstances live (in vivo) instruction may be more suitable. Or, you may wish to start instruction with a different tool, such as premade

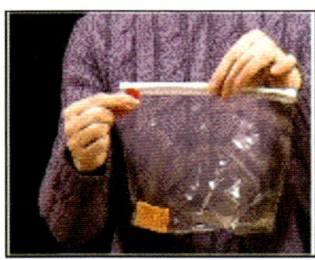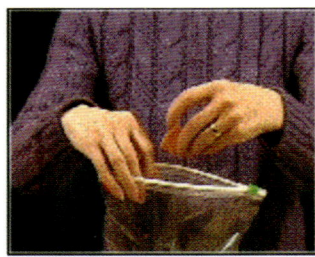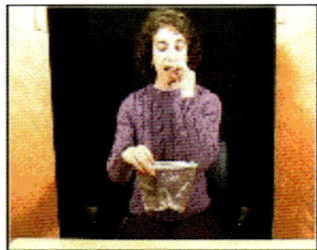

Figure 6–2. Example of a sequence of scene cues for acting out "opening a bag of crackers."

scene cues. It is important to note, however, that a limitation of beginning instruction with premade scene cues is the likelihood that three to five scene cues may not be enough to capture the critical information needed for the learner to reconstruct the task. In this case, more scene cues to capture critical steps may need to be added.

Premade Scene Cues

With premade scene cues, the learner works on routines on the tabletop without benefit of the computer video clips, which encourages learning from symbolic images rather than a reenactment of the routine. Premade scene cues can be used to work on the same routines as in the previous exercise, or slightly more complex routines.

Goals: concept development (gestalt form):
- To capture familiar experiences
- To direct attention to the sequence of the routines
- To make the routines predictable.

Modes: Visual Instructional Mode (VIM), Visual Expressive Mode (VEM)

Materials:
- photos of critical steps of routine
- photos of steps from other routines, for use as foils
- "sequence display"—this is a rectangular display onto which the photos are affixed in the proper order (you will need to have two copies of each photo)
- actual objects used in routine.

Example: Toothbrushing
Prepare three premade scene cues, such as separate pictures of a boy holding toothpaste and a toothbrush, a boy squeezing toothpaste onto the toothbrush, and a boy putting the toothbrush in his mouth.

Step 1: Show the learner the three pictures in the proper sequence on the table, and display the sequence strip (Figure 6–3A).

Step 2: Model the three steps of the routine for the learner.

Step 3: Mix up the order of the three photos on the table, and direct the learner to match each photo on the table to the identical photo on the picture strip.

Step 4: Mix up the order of the three photos on the table and place the picture strip out of the learner's view (e.g., in a box). Direct the learner to put the three photos in the correct order.

Step 5: On one side of the table, place the first two photos in the sequence. On the other side of the table, place the third photo amid two foils (e.g., a picture of a boy brushing his hair and a picture of a boy petting a dog). Point out the first two photos in the sequence and direct the learner to pick the photo that completes the sequence (Figure 6–3B).

Step 6: Ask the learner (through speech or visual directives) to perform the routine. If he cannot, encourage him to look at the photos and the sequence strip for reference. Although this may seem like a setback, it is actually an important part of instruction, as it shows the learner he can use visuals to assist his memory.

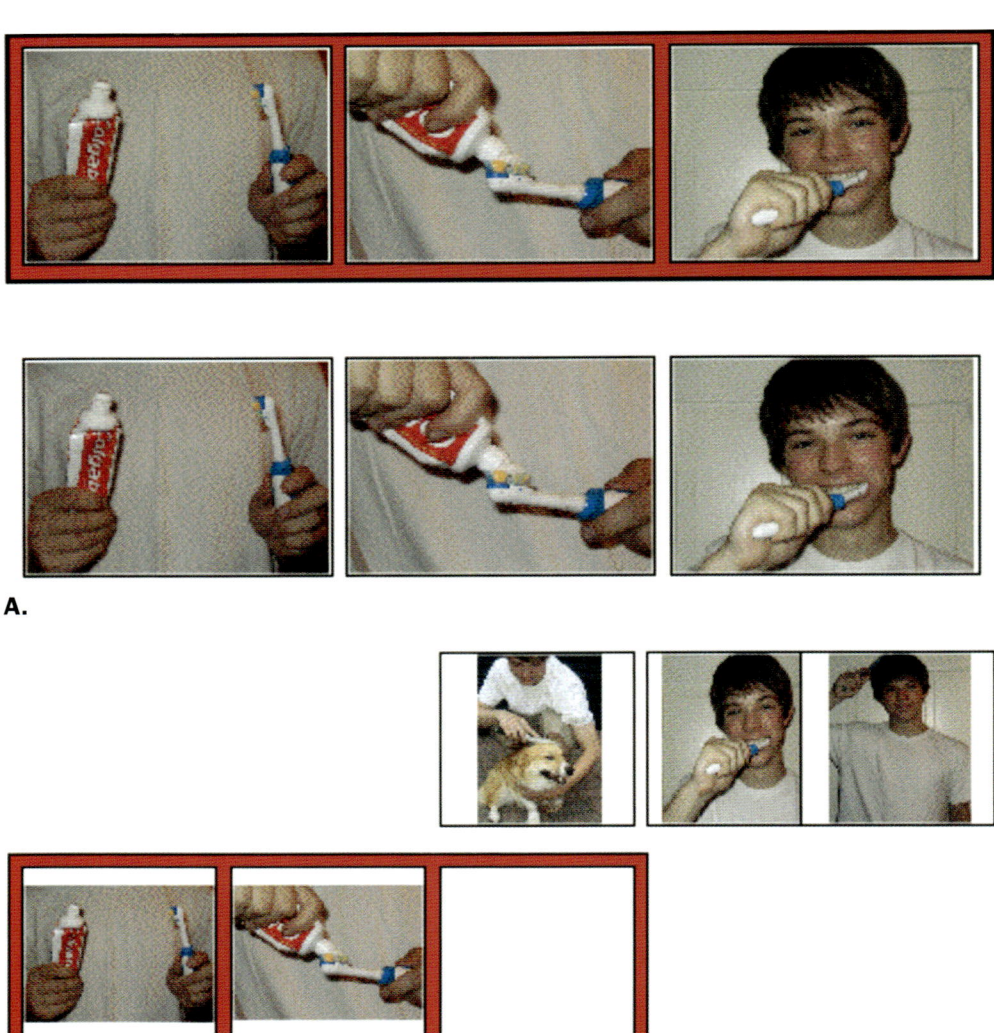

Figure 6–3. A. Example of a sequence of scene cues for acting out "toothbrushing" (match to sample). **B.** Example of a sequence completion activity with foils.

Step 7: Review the photos on the table and the sequence strip. For a short time (5 to 10 seconds), perform a competing activity (e.g., get up to open the door, comment on the learner's clothing, etc.). Ask the learner to perform the routine. This imposed latency is designed to develop the learner's ability to maintain a task over time.

Step 8: Encourage the learner to perform the sequence independently and with minimum assistance of scene cues, repeating earlier steps if necessary.

This type of activity is effective for numerous moderately complex routines, such as washing hands, getting dressed or preparing a snack from the refrigerator, and so forth.

Buildable Scene Cues and Whole Scene Displays

Once the learner demonstrates competence with learning routines from premade scene cues, you can introduce buildable scene cues and whole scene displays. Again, this moves the learner toward more analytical thinking and broader use of language.

Goals:
- To provide visual supports to perform activities
- To help the learner make successful transitions between activities
- To develop the learner's understanding of the six types of element cues and then lay further groundwork for using elements to create an understanding of whole concepts (gestalt form and analytical processing).

Materials:
- whole scene display of an environment
- photos of objects (object elements with background removed) from the whole scene environment
- objects from the whole scene environment.

Modes: VIM, VEM, VOM

Buildable scene cues and whole scene displays can be used for performing routines, preparing for them, and transitioning between them.

Performance of Routines

Example: Buttering toast.

Step 1: Using the object element photos with the backgrounds removed, show the learner how to put the toast on top of the plate and the butter on top of the toast

Step 2: Reconstruct the sequence by reenacting the routine for the learner and modeling how to butter an actual piece of toast. Direct the learner (through speech and with appropriate visuals) to do so (Figures 6–4A and 6–4B).

Along with teaching the learner this routine, this type of exercise helps him become familiar with additional language elements such as prepositions (butter *on* the toast) and provides a structured opportunity to interpret embedded actions (*spreading* butter is learned by viewing the activity as well as acting out the activity). This exercise is also appropriate for any activity that has a goal-oriented sequence of steps, such as brushing teeth, pouring a drink, or getting ready for a bath.

Transitions

Visual schedules are typically used to help learners with ASD understand transitions. We offer the following approach as an alternative, which we believe provides a richer contextual understanding. Furthermore, it promotes the opportunity for information to be shared and a conversation to occur between the learner and his communication partner.

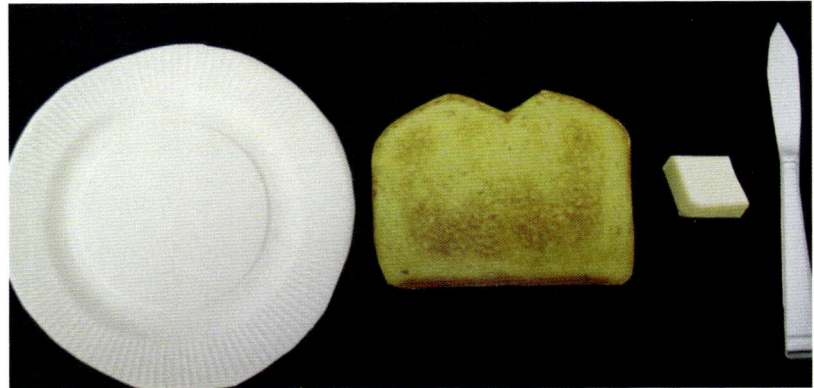

A.

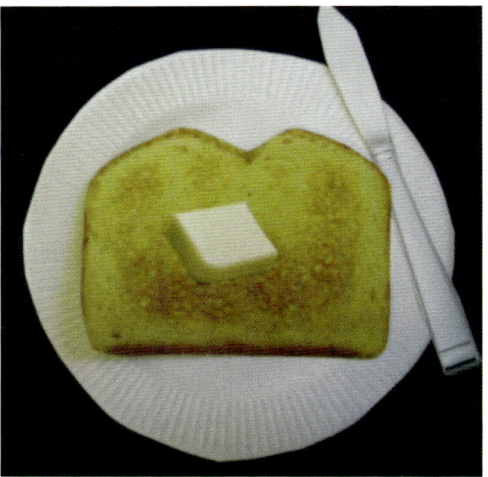

B.

Figure 6–4. A. Object elements (photographs with background removed) of materials used for teaching buttering toast. **B.** Buildable scene using object elements (with backgrounds removed) for teaching buttering toast.

Example: Directing the child to get up from the kitchen table and go to the bathroom:

Step 1: Sitting at a table, present the learner with whole scene displays of the current rooms (e.g., the kitchen and the bathroom).

Step 2: Place a photo of the learner with the background removed on the whole scene of the kitchen.

Step 3: Pick up the photo of the learner and place it on the whole scene of the bathroom while saying, "Go to the bathroom."

Step 4: Walk with the learner to the bathroom.

Step 5: Repeat the exercise, encouraging the learner to walk to the bathroom without your guidance.

Once the individual learns to follow directives, this type of exercise can also be used to show him how to request and protest as the need arises. For example, when the learner wants to express that he would like to use the bathroom, he can move his picture from the kitchen whole scene to the bathroom whole scene. If you direct him to go use the bathroom but he does not want to go, he can remove the picture from the bathroom whole scene and place it on a more preferred whole scene. It may take several repetitions of this exercise, but once learners become familiar with using whole scenes in this fashion, many become adept at using them to request and protest during daily life.

Preparation

Whole scenes can be used to prepare for an activity, such as getting ready for a bath. This exercise can be done at home, in preparation for an actual bath, or in a school environment or clinic, where the instructor prepares the material and advises the parent on how to carry out the activity out at home.

In the bathroom the parent and the learner place object element cues (such as a towel, soap, shampoo, a rubber duck, and other toys) with the backgrounds removed on the whole scene of the bathroom (Figure 6–5). By putting the symbols on or off the whole scene display, the learner can respond to directives, such as "go get your towel" (parent places towel on the display); make requests, such as "I want my rubber duck" (learner places rubber duck on display); and indicate protests, such as "I don't want to take a bath" (learner removes his picture from the display).

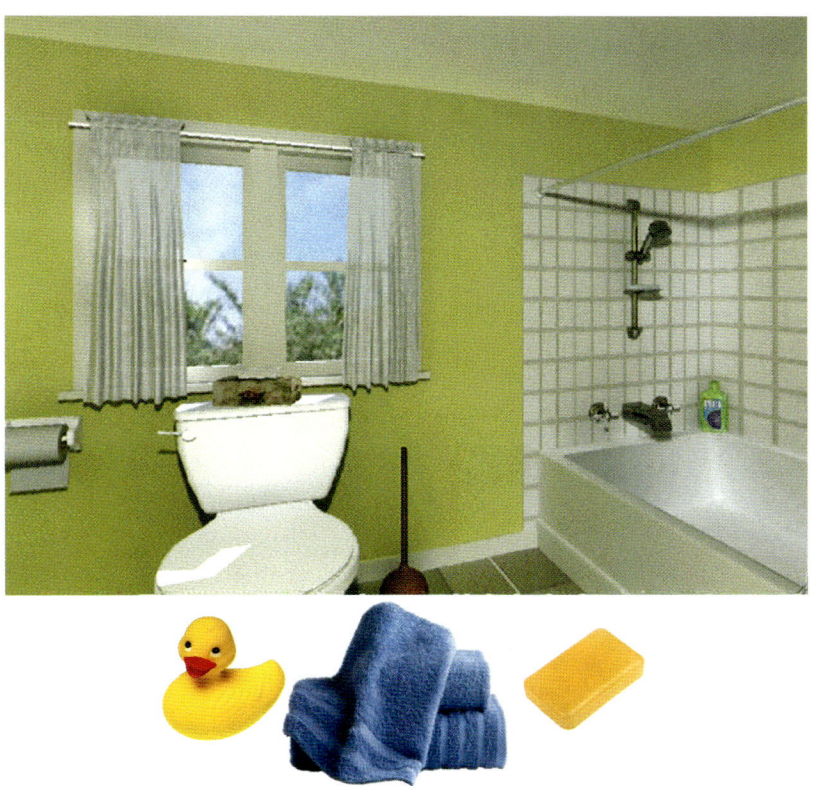

Figure 6–5. Example of a whole scene display with object elements cues (for preparation for a bath).

The exchange can go back and forth while interacting with the element cues and the actual items.

This exercise can be used for preparing for any activity, such as getting ready for school, a trip to the library, or a visit to a friend or relative's home.

Mixed Displays

Mixed displays can be used as a bridge between whole scenes displays (which are contextualized) and conversation displays (which are not).

Goal: To promote analytical processing and expression.

Materials:
- buildable whole scene display with message window to hold element cues
- object element cues, such as a ball, a car, and a dog
- agent element cues, such as a boy and a neighbor
- action element cues, such as running, kicking, and petting
- spatial element cues, such as on, in, and under
- attribute element cues, such as big, small, red, and happy,

Modes: VIM, VEM

Example: View of the front of the learner's house.

Work with the learner to create scene cues with the element cues, placing them on the whole scene and in a message window under the scene. Initially, the instructor models the construction of the scene. This combination of the gestalt of the scene display and element

captioning helps the learner recognize the semantic relationships between and among the visual symbols as they relate to a recognizable and comprehensible experience.

Depending on the learner's comprehension level, a variety of language skills can be emphasized. For example:

- a scene cue of "the neighbor is brushing the dog" shows the learner how to interpret element symbols linking an actor (the neighbor), an action (brushing), and the recipient of the action (the dog) (Figure 6–6).

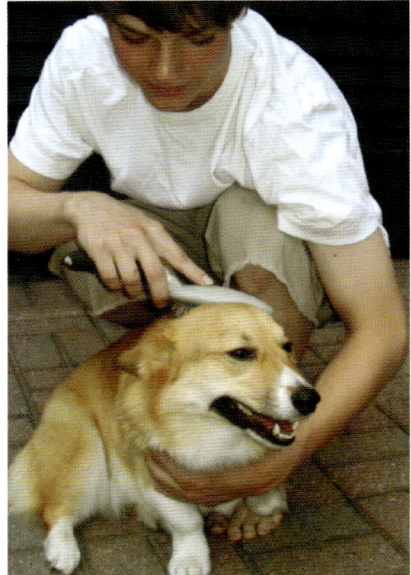

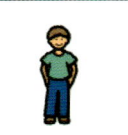  

Figure 6–6. Mixed scene display depicting "boy brushes dog." (From The Picture Communication Symbols ©1981–2007 by Mayer-Johnson LLC. All Rights Reserved Worldwide. Used with permission.)

- a scene cue of "the boy gets in the car" shows the learner how to interpret symbols for prepositions embedded within action verbs
- emphasizing specific aspects of scene cues (e.g., the red car, the small dog, the happy neighbor) shows the learner how to interpret symbols for adjectives embedded within nouns.

Conversation Displays

Conversation displays are used to display a series of symbols relating to a single topic of interest to the learner. Unlike whole scenes, conversation displays must be processed analytically—the learner views each element one at a time and gradually gains meaning from the larger display based on his ability to act on his understanding of the semantic relationships between each element (i.e., agent/action/object) and the display's syntactic structure.

Tabletop and Natural Environment Activities

Conversation displays can be used to enhance comprehension and expression by specifically teaching and encouraging language use through structured, explicit instruction on the tabletop or through implicit instruction in the natural environment where the need for structured training is minimized. They can in effect become a mobile language display providing situational opportunities for visual language practice. The goal is not for the learner to immediately repeat or imitate a targeted phrase or action, but rather to allow him to observe how language use can affect his environment. By observing behavior and having the opportunity to see the visual language elements that support that action, the learner may internalize the semantic and syntactic relationships among the symbols mapped to the behavior.

When creating conversation displays in the natural environment:

- Make sure word order reflects spoken English (e.g., agent, action, object).
- Place vocabulary that is often repeated across multiple displays/pages in a consistent location on each display, supporting automaticity in accessing that vocabulary.
- Provide consistent and repeated exposure to the communication displays.

Comprehension

Goal: To enhance comprehension.

Materials:
- materials that make up a preferred activity
- element cues from that preferred activity.

Mode: VIM

Preparation and delivery of this intervention should include these steps[3]:

Step 1: Generate a list of preferred routines and activities the learner engages in (e.g., blowing bubbles, playing with toy trains, etc.).

---

[3]This lesson is adapted from *Engineering the Preschool Environment for Interactive Symbolic Communication* by Carol Goosens, Sharon Sapp Crain, and Pamela Elder. Southeast Augmentative Communication Conference Publications, 1992.

Step 2: Order the list based on the learner's motivation to participate and how often the activity occurs.

Step 3: List all the possible vocabulary associated with a specific activity (e.g., nouns, verbs, adjectives, prepositions, and comments such as "I like that!" or "That's yucky!").

Step 4: Create a conversation display.

Step 5: Prominently place conversation displays in locations where they will be used.

Step 6: Present the display pertaining to that activity during the preferred activity (e.g., blowing bubbles, playing with toy trains). The learner's communication partner should place symbols within the message window while speaking (e.g., "I'm blowing big bubbles!" or "The train is going fast!").

Step 7: Use these displays regularly during activities the learner enjoys, increasing the likelihood that he will internalize linguistic rules for symbolic communication use.

Expression
Conversation displays can also be used in the natural environment to improve learners' ability to express themselves.

Goal: To improve expression skills.

Materials: Same as above.

Mode: VEM

These conversation displays should include elements that represent various parts of speech, including agents (e.g., the learner, parents, siblings, classmates, etc.), actions (e.g., verbs), prepositions, and modifiers (e.g., adjectives). These displays can be used to help learners use a wider vocabulary range and communicate for more pragmatic purposes (e.g., commenting, directing).

The instructor can create these displays by using photographs and graphics such as Mayer-Johnson symbols that depict preferred activities (e.g., swimming, movies), depending on the level of representation the learner comprehends. Displays might initially contain only the agent, action, and object, and additional vocabulary (e.g., prepositions, adjectives, etc.) can be added as the learner becomes successful using the display. While using this type of display, you should describe the learners' actions to model symbol use.

Symbols on the display should be arranged in columns, from left to right, as follows: agents, actions, modifiers/prepositions, and objects. The symbols should be removable, and a sentence strip with a message window should be located at the top of the display. This gives the learner a static visual representation of sentence creation. These displays may also be used to enhance the linguistic complexity of the learner's message (e.g., if the learner recognizes the symbol for "bubble," the adult can add "blow" and "big" to create "blow a big bubble").

Figures 6-7A, 6-7B, and 6-7C are examples of a conversational display using Mayer-Johnson and digital symbols. We recommend using a color-coding system to promote visual organization of the displays. A suggested color code is offered in Table 6-1.

In addition, miscellaneous words such as "wh" words (who, what, when, where), exclamations (uh-oh, wow), negative words (no, don't), and pronouns/people (I, you) can be coded purple.

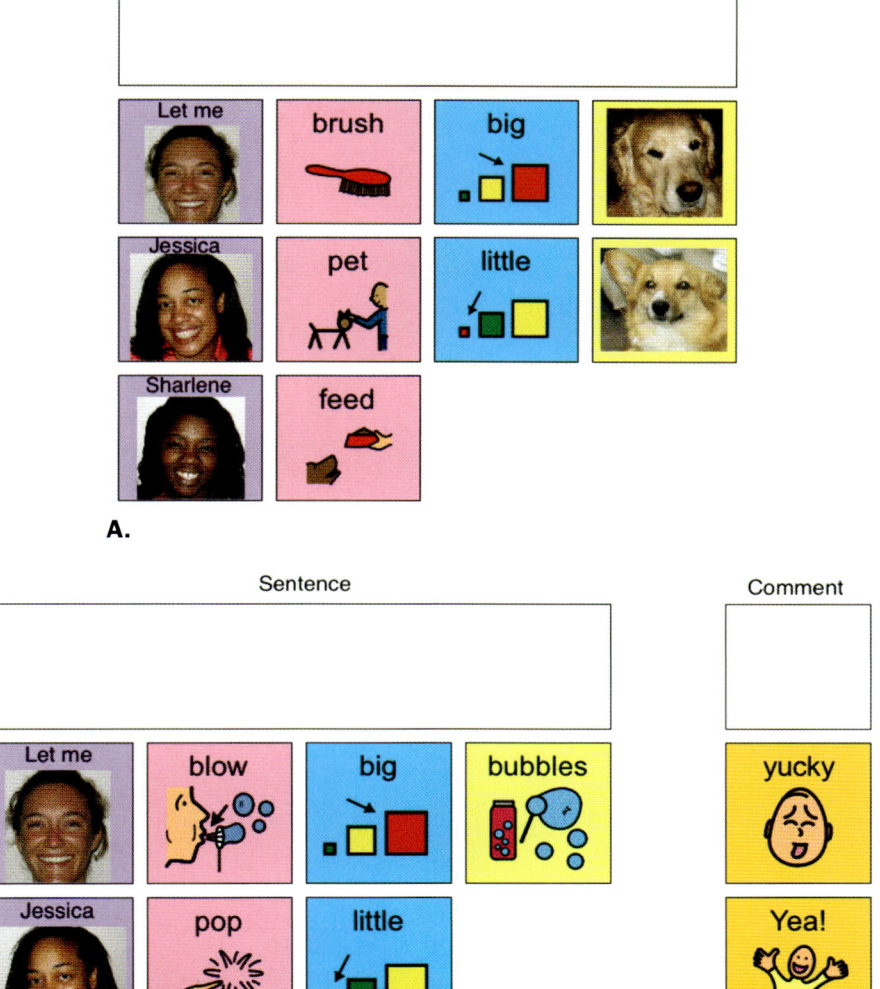

A.

Sentence

Comment

B.

Figure 6–7. A. Conversational display with multiple agents for feeding/grooming dogs of different sizes. (From The Picture Communication Symbols ©1981–2007 by Mayer-Johnson LLC. All Rights Reserved Worldwide. Used with permission.) **B.** Conversational display with multiple agents for bubbles activity. (From The Picture Communication Symbols ©1981-2007 by Mayer-Johnson LLC. All Rights Reserved Worldwide. Used with permission.) *continues*

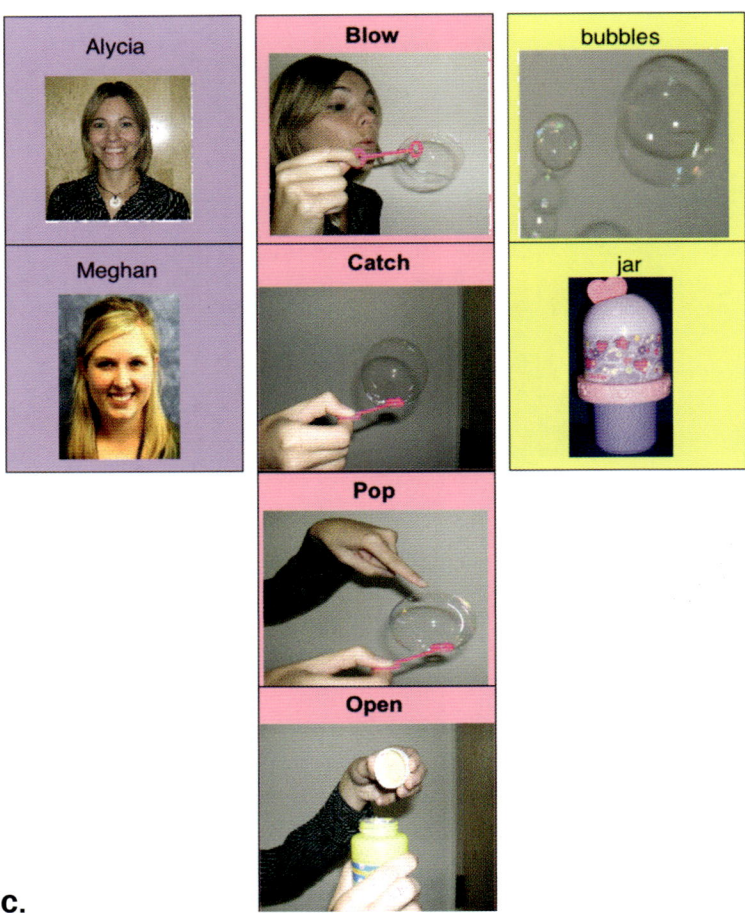

C.

Figure 6–7. *continued* **C.** Conversational display with multiple agents for bubbles activity (using digital photographs only)

Table 6–1. Suggested Color Codes

Word Category	Example	Color
Agents	Me, Bob	purple
Verbs	come, open	pink
Descriptors (adjectives and adverbs)	pretty, slow	blue
Prepositions	in, off	green
Nouns	car, string	Yellow
Comments	Yay, yucky	orange

Language Expansion Activities

The next component is language expansion, which includes activities for vocabulary development and use of directives and reminders.

Tabletop Activities for Vocabulary Development

A series of tabletop activities using element cues can be used to expand the learner's visual representative vocabulary. In addition to teaching the learner new words, instruction aims to show him their relationship to other words and concepts, so he can recognize and use the new words in multiple contexts. Words can be selected from the Experiential Knowledge Profile environment vocabulary list to ensure that vocabulary items are relevant to the learner's daily experience (see Appendix C).

Materials: Relevant element cues.

Modes: VIM, VEM

Identical Matching

The first exercise matches object element cues to identical object element cues at the same level of representation (Figure 6–8). For example, lay out four photos of animals on one side of the table (e.g., a dog, a cat, a pig, and a monkey), and the same photos on the other side of the table. Provide the learner with sufficient support to accurately complete the activity of matching the photographs of the animals. Once the learner can complete this exercise with photo-

graphs, repeat the exercise with more abstract representations, such as colored or line drawings (without mingling different levels of representation).

Matching Multiple Exemplars

The next exercise matches multiple examples of object element cues that are at the same level of representation but are not identical. For example, lay out 10 photos of household objects, 5 of which are the same object (such as a toothbrush) but in different colors or sizes. While providing the learner with sufficient support to complete the activity, direct him to match the five toothbrush photos to the real object (Figure 6–9).

Expansion of Representational Understanding

Next, work with the learner to match object element cues from different levels of representation. Begin with two levels, such as photos and pictures. For example, mix up a display of 10 element cues of household objects, such as photos and colored drawings of combs, toothbrushes,

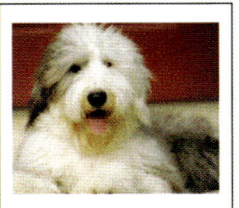 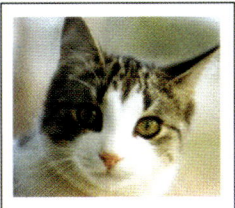 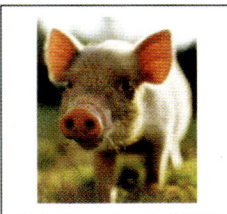 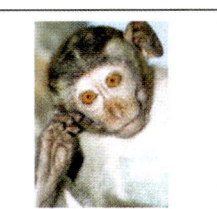

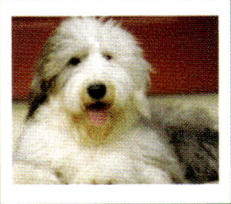

Figure 6–8. Example of an identical matching task (match photographs of dogs).

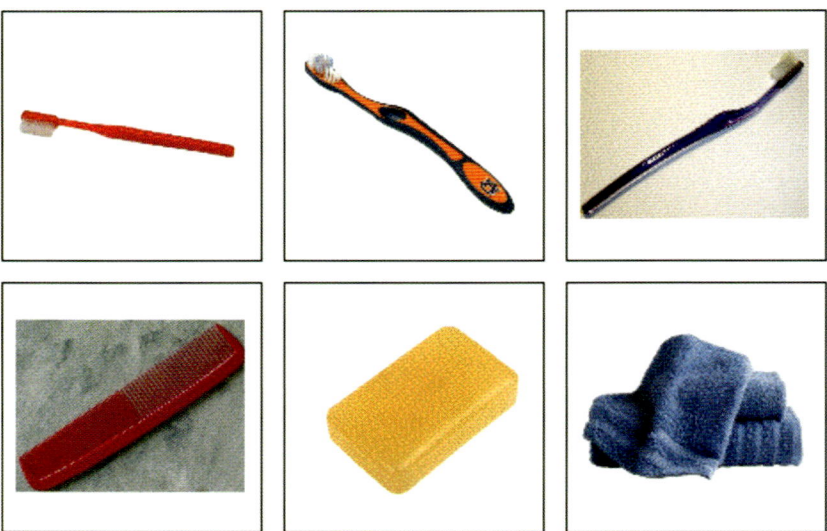

Figure 6–9. Example of matching activity using multiple exemplars with foils (match to object toothbrush).

hair brushes, bars of soap, and cups. Provide the learner with sufficient support to accurately complete the activity and direct him to match the different levels of representation of the object element cues. (Figure 6–10).

Once the learner can successfully complete this task with two levels of representation, additional levels can be added, such as line drawings, and, for more advanced learners, text.

Categorical Understanding

Next, work on enhancing the learner's understanding of the function or class of similar items—what is known as categorical understanding. For example, work with the learner to indicate all the birds among a display of photos of animals, all the shirts among a display of drawings of clothing, and so forth. Consider beginning with a single level of representation and then use multiple levels simultaneously.

Once the learner becomes competent with these categorical matching exercises, introduce exercises that focus on expanding vocabulary (Figure 6–11). Exercises developed by Beck, McKeown, and Kucan for developing spoken language vocabulary suggest initially emphasizing words with great instructional potential (Beck et al., 2002). This principle can also be applied when working with learners with ASD. For example, the word cup is a good choice as the basis of a vocabulary expansion task because it can be used in multiple environments (e.g., kitchen, bathroom, at school, on a picnic), and it can be connected to various verbs (drink, sip), nouns (juice, milk), and adjectives (plastic, glass, big, and little).

To increase noun vocabulary, it is wise to initially introduce the most frequently used and familiar item in a categorical class and then progress toward expansion to less frequently used vocab-

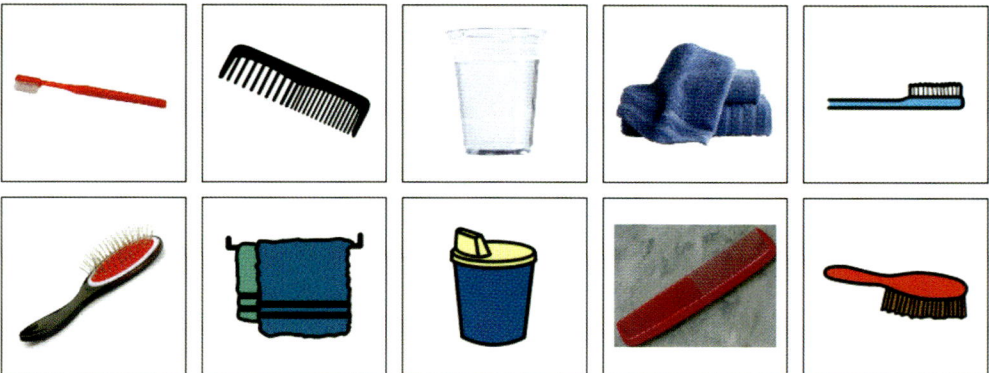

Figure 6–10. Example of expansion of representational understanding (match photographs to different levels of representation). (From The Picture Communication Symbols ©1981–2007 by Mayer-Johnson LLC. All Rights Reserved Worldwide. Used with permission.)

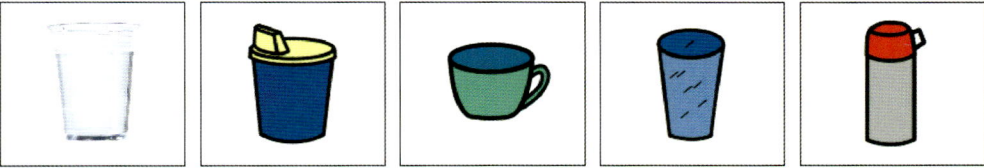

Figure 6–11. Example of vocabulary expansion activity for items used for drinking. (From The Picture Communication Symbols ©1981–2007 by Mayer-Johnson LLC. All Rights Reserved Worldwide. Used with permission.)

ulary. For example when introducing visual symbols that represent drinking implements, first present a visual symbol of a cup, as it is likely to be the most familiar and frequently used item within the categorical class. Once the learner has demonstrated his competency with the symbol for cup, introduce less frequently occurring objects within the same categorical class such as mug or a thermos.

Step 1: Show the learner a plastic cup and mime how you drink from it.

Step 2: Display five drinking implements, such as a plastic cup, a glass, a bottle, a mug, and a thermos. Demonstrate that all these objects are used for drinking.

Step 3: Mix in objects not used for drinking (a bowl, a toaster, a fork, etc.).

Step 4: Provide the learner with sufficient support to accurately complete the activity. Direct the learner to choose the objects used for drinking by demonstrating their function. Adding a beverage to the drinking implements may be helpful to the learner's understanding of the task.

Environment Sorting

Next, work with the learner to match element cues to their appropriate environment (Figure 6-12).

Step 1: Display two common whole scenes, such as large photos of a bathroom and a kitchen.

Step 2: Display a mix of 10 object element cues from both scenes (photos or drawings of a toothbrush, toothpaste, soap, a refrigerator, a bottle of juice, a toaster, etc.).

Step 3: Provide the learner with sufficient support to accurately complete the activity of matching the element cues to the appropriate environment.

While working on these exercises, a symbol-rich environment should be simultaneously created for the learner, demonstrating how the object elements from the tabletop appear in the natural environment. A symbol-rich environment also sets the stage for the exercises described in the section that follows on directives and reminders.

An important first step is deciding on a list of relevant and functional objects to associate with visual cues.

It is pedagogically sound to focus initially on the objects and people the learner interacts with most. At school, examples might include the desk, classmates, the blackboard, and the classroom hamster. At home, examples might include the refrigerator, doors, television, the DVD player, the family pet, family members and preferred foods and toys. You should also pick some quirky objects that, for whatever reason, hold the learner's interest. Keep in mind it is not

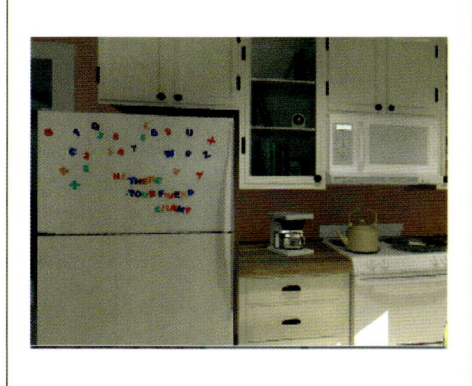
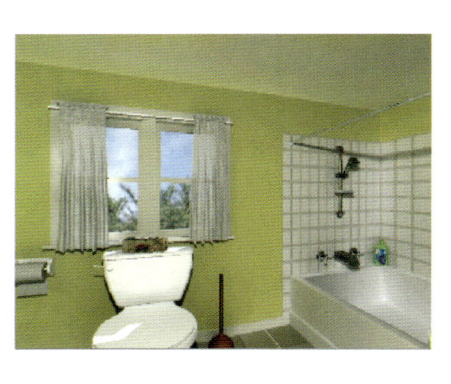

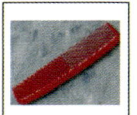
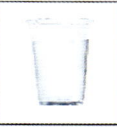
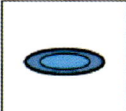
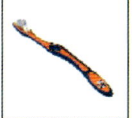
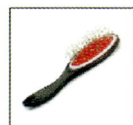
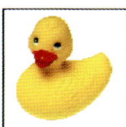

Figure 6–12. Example of environment sorting activity (kitchen and bathroom). (From The Picture Communication Symbols ©1981–2007 by Mayer-Johnson LLC. All Rights Reserved Worldwide. Used with permission.)

necessary nor recommended to label every object in the environment, as this may only overwhelm the learner. It is more effective to start with a limited number and gradually introduce new object labels.

For the items selected, the relevant visual symbols should be placed in a prominent location. Symbols for objects can be affixed to the actual objects or placed nearby. Symbols for people can be temporarily held by a person. Because it is not always feasible to leave all the symbols in place, it may be helpful to store them where they can be easily accessed. It is important to have the visual symbols logistically available in order to seize opportune moments to use them when communicating with the learner.

Directives and Reminders

Element cues can be used in relevant situations as they arise to improve the learner's ability to interact with other people, and as a mechanism to improve generalization to novel environments. Element cues are used as a retrieval mechanism to help the learner see the relevance between what he has learned and the current situation, as in the following exercises.

> **Goal:** To help the learner follow directions, comment on his behavior, or activate knowledge of a prior experience.
>
> **Mode:** VIM
>
> **Materials**: Relevant element cues.

Single Element Cues

In anticipation of an activity, show the learner a single object element cue

designed to activate his memory of a sequence of events about to unfold (Figure 6–13). For example, when the learner is about is about to visit grandmother, display her photo. When he is about to go home from school, show him an image of a school bus.

Combined Element Cues

Use combined element cues, such as an object element cue and an action element cue, to give the learner instruction or comment on his behavior (Figure 6–14). For example, prior to directing the learner to drink a glass of milk, display

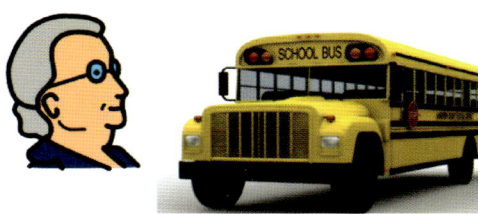

Figure 6–13. Example of use of agent and object element cues used to prepare for upcoming activities.

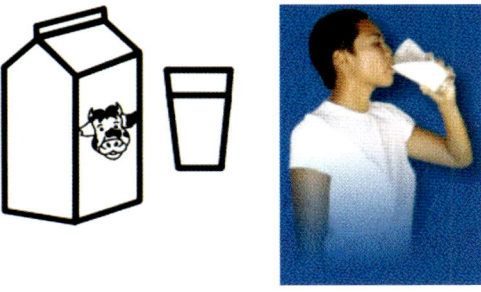

Figure 6–14. Example of object element cue and scene cue used to direct (From The Picture Communication Symbols ©1981–2007 by Mayer-Johnson LLC. All Rights Reserved Worldwide. Used with permission.)

the symbol of the action of drinking and another symbol that depicts milk. To comment on his behavior, point to the image of the learner and an action element that symbolizes drinking (i.e., "learner" is drinking his milk).

Temporal Displays

The next component is temporal displays, which help the learner understand time-related aspects of learning, such as how much time remains in an activity, how many trials are needed to complete a task, what the reinforcement is for completing a specified activity, and when he can expect to receive a reinforcement. Note that visual timers are used to refer to the passage of time *within* an activity. By contrast, visual schedules refer to one activity *in relation* to another.

There are three types of temporal displays: visual timers, countdown displays, and first/then displays. The following exercises are designed to introduce each display type to learners. Once you do this, temporal displays can be integrated into the exercises described earlier in this chapter. Temporal displays are included as part of the Visual Organization Mode (VOM).

Visual Timers

A range of visual timers can be used, including digital and analog clocks, stopwatches, hourglass timers, and the Time Timer™ device, to depict the passage of time. Their function is to show the learner how much time has passed or how much time is left before an activity ends. This is important whether the learner has positive or negative feelings about the activity. If it is an activity he enjoys (a preferred activity), the timer makes the ending less of a surprise, so he is less likely to get upset. If it is an activity he dislikes (a nonpreferred activity), the timer shows him there is only so much time remaining before he can switch to a more preferred activity.

Seek out visual timers likely to be understood by the learner,. The learner needs to develop an appreciation that the visual timer represents the passage of time and understand the relationship of the visual timer to an activity's beginning or end.

Materials:
- visual timer
- photos of visual timers set to start and end at specific times
- materials for an activity the learner enjoys and can do with the timer nearby, such as a puzzle.

Example: Time Timer™ (Figure 6–15)

Step 1: Set the Time Timer™ to the determined amount of elapsed time for the activity, such as 10 minutes.

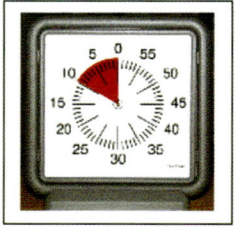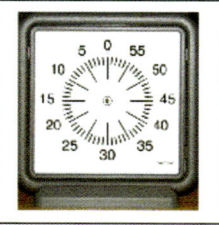

Figure 6–15. Example of the Time Timer™. (Time Timer™ Images used with permission from Time Timer LLC.)

Step 2: Show the learner a photo of the Time Timer™ with 10 minutes and a photo of the visual timer with the time elapsed.

Step 3: Start the Time Timer™.

Step 4: Work with the learner on the puzzle, occasionally directing his attention to the Time Timer™ and pointing out how much time remains.

Step 5: When time runs out, point out that the Time Timer™ now looks like the second photo.

Once the learner is familiar with visual timers, you can use them whenever engaging in a task or activity with a fixed start and end time.

Countdown Displays

Countdown displays help the learner understand the number of trials or specific tasks he has to complete within an activity. There are many types—for complex exercises with a large number of tasks you may want to use a board with a linear display of removable items, such as tokens, rings, or appealing photographs. For exercises with five or less tasks, you can use your hand, counting down one finger at a time. You can also create reward displays in which you present a certain amount of a desired item (e.g., pistachio nuts or baseball cards) and allow the learner to take one for every correct answer.

Materials:
- countdown board set up with items corresponding to the number of tasks or trials within the activity
- a task with a fixed number of trials, such as a matching exercise.

Example: Countdown board with tokens (Figure 6–16).

Step 1: Lay out 20 photos that include 10 pairs (i.e., two dogs, two cats, two horses, two monkeys, etc.).

Step 2: Direct the learner to pick out matching pairs and place them in a box.

Step 3: Each time the learner picks out a correct pair, give him a token. Repeat until all 10 tokens are removed from the board.

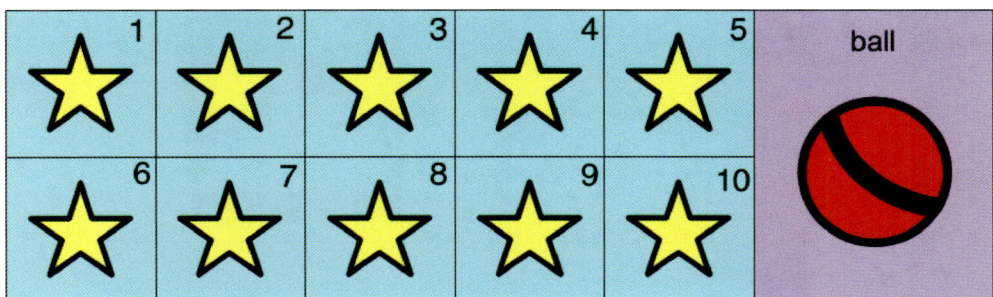

Figure 6–16. Example of countdown board with reinforcement. (From The Picture Communication Symbols ©1981–2007 by Mayer-Johnson LLC. All Rights Reserved Worldwide. Used with permission.)

First/Then Displays

First/then displays help the learner anticipate what activity will follow the completion of another—most often a preferred activity or reward follows a less preferred activity. First/then displays typically show a visual representing the first activity on the left side and a visual representing the subsequent activity or reward on the right side (Figure 6–17).

Materials:
- blank first/then display with left column labeled "first" and right column labeled "then"
- photos representing preferred and nonpreferred activities
- materials for preferred and nonpreferred activities.

Example: Playing video game as reward for completing matching task.

Step 1: Display photos representing a video game and a matching task. A screen shot of the video game might represent the game and a photo of a montage of three photos might represent the matching task.

Step 2: Pointing to the appropriate photo, say, "First we'll do this, then you can do this."

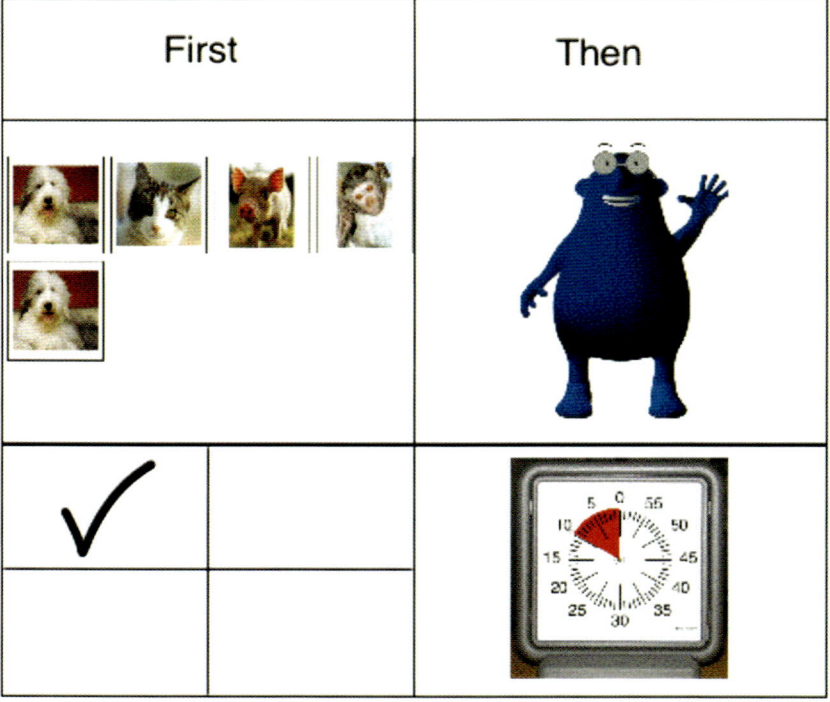

Figure 6–17. Example of first/then display expanded to include number of trials and/or duration of each activity. (From The Picture Communication Symbols ©1981–2007 by Mayer-Johnson LLC. All Rights Reserved Worldwide. Used with permission. Time Timer™ Images used with permission from Time Timer LLC.)

Step 3: Repeat Step 2, this time placing the photos on the first/then display.

Step 4: Direct the learner to complete the matching task.

Step 5: Allow the learner to play the video game.

The embedding of the first/then concept with the time element and the number of trials was developed in the Autism Language Program at Children's Hospital Boston and is being used successfully with many children with autism. We have found that, once the learner grasps the first/then display concept, it can be used effectively in combination with countdown displays and visual timers. As an example, consider creating a first/then display showing the learner that if he solves 10 math problems he can play a video game for 5 minutes. Each time the learner gives a correct answer, check off a countdown box on the "first" side of the display. Once he gives 10 correct answers, he can play the video game for the 5 minutes of designated time set on the Time Timer™. The clarity provided by embedding the number of trials and duration with the concept of first/then can have a profound effect on successful task completion and behavior management.

References

Beck., I. L., McKeown, M. G., & Kucan, L. (2002). *Bringing words to life. Robust vocabulary instruction.* New York: The Guilford Press.

Shane, H. C., & Alpert, P. (2005, November). *Electronic screen media for persons with Autism Spectrum Disorders.* Presentation at the annual meeting of the American Speech-Language-Hearing Association; Philadelphia.

Vygotsky, L. S. (1962). *Thought and language* (F. Hanfmann & G. Valar, Trans.) Cambridge, MA: MIT Press.

7

Special Considerations

In this chapter, we discuss a number of issues relevant to the VIP that exceed the scope of the previous six chapters:

- controlling inappropriate behavior
- expression of pain and discomfort
- the inclusive classroom
- using visuals inside and outside the home
- intervention for Pre-Level 1 learners
- intervention for learners who read
- selecting appropriate assistive technology.

Controlling Inappropriate Behavior

Responding effectively to behavior problems is a critical part of working with learners with ASD. Many individuals are prone to outbursts and meltdowns, and some may lash out at other people or hurt themselves.

Behavioral and pharmacologic approaches are commonly used to control such behavior. Functional Behavioral Analysis is a popular method that aims to identify and address triggers and consequences of inappropriate behavior. Parents frequently ask for, and physicians often prescribe, medication to reduce anxiety, address behavioral issues associated with ASD, and to calm the learner. Although both approaches can be effective, we propose that the VIP can also play a major role in controlling inappropriate behavior for the simple reason that communication failure is often at the root of behavior problems, and the VIP enables learners to communicate more effectively. In some cases, the effective use of visuals may preclude the need to use medication. The following are some areas where the VIP can reduce inappropriate behavior as a result of improved communication.

Poor Requesting Skills

Many tantrums result from a learner's inability to communicate what he wants, whether it is an object (a drink of water, a snack, a toy, etc.) or an action (to play a game, go outside, use the bathroom, etc.). Individuals who learn to use element and scene cues and conversation displays can become effective requesters, making them less likely to get frustrated and act out.

Acting Out as an Escape Behavior

When a learner with ASD acts out, a commonly imposed strategy is to remove him from the situation, often referred to as giving him a time-out. The problem is that in many cases, a time-out is exactly what he wants—that is, he wishes to be left alone or to escape a nonpreferred task—so he acts out to get one. In such instances, the time-out provides inadvertent reinforcement, encouraging him to continue to misbehave whenever he wants to escape from an unpleasant activity or experience.

Appropriate visuals can be used to help break this cycle: Teach the learner how to express his desire for a break and he no longer needs to act out when he wants one. For example, he can be taught to use a simple hand gesture or an element cue, such as a gesture for "break" or "stop" or an element cue such as a picture of his bedroom. If the learner repeatedly asks for breaks and this presents a problem, you may need to place limits on the number of breaks per day. This can be represented visually by checking off a predetermined number of break boxes or by giving the learner a set number of break pictures to use each day. Another effective strategy is to teach the learner to specify an alternative to the undesirable event or activity.

Attention Seeking

Conversely, a learner may act out when he wants attention. Again, teaching the hand gesture for "help" and showing him how to use visuals to ask for another person's attention (such as using a picture of the person whose attention he desires) can be helpful here. A visual timer can help the learner understand how much time the person can spend with him before returning to another activity or how long he must wait before he can receive the attention he seeks.

Transition Problems

Tantrums often result from a learner's failure to understand that he needs to move from one setting to another and he needs to understand that an activity will terminate. He may be disappointed at the abrupt end of a preferred activity, fail to understand that a nonpreferred activity will soon end, or be unable to anticipate the sequence of events at school or on an outing.

Visual supports are often effective in reducing inappropriate behavior that results from such scenarios. For example, using your fingers to indicate that the learner can go down the slide three more times (a form of countdown) or a visual timer to show he can watch a video for 5 more minutes makes the activity's end less startling.

Language Comprehension Problems

Inappropriate behavior often occurs when a learner does not know what is expected of him because he does not comprehend instructions or requests or is confused in general by speech directed to him. A useful strategy is the effective use of VIM. When instructors and parents use relevant visuals to support spoken language, there is often a marked behavior improvement. For example, showing pictures of the family car and Aunt Beth as you say, "We are going to visit Aunt Beth" provides an explanation for the trip, easing the transition into the car.

Coping with Surprises

Unforeseen events are often upsetting for learners with ASD, especially if they cannot understand the reason for a sudden change of plans. These two examples, from actual experiences related by parents, are typical:

■ Timothy happily accompanied his mother to the town library on a clear fall day—a setting he enjoyed because of his almost obsessive interest in books. Unfortunately, he was disappointed to find the library doors closed because the librarian was away for the day. Without warning, Timothy punched his mother, knocking her to the ground, and then began to strike his head against a granite curbstone repeatedly.

■ Darrin was enjoying a leisurely Saturday with his family during a severe lightning and thunderstorm. He was unaffected by the raging storm until it knocked out electrical power. For hours his parents and siblings were unable to explain why the lights, television, or computer games were not working. Darrin grew increasingly agitated as the afternoon wore on, and his behavior worsened in the evening because of his long-time fear of darkness.

Although such events are unforeseeable, you can use visuals to teach effective coping strategies. We recommend preparing a lesson that shows a visual schedule in the traditional linear format (Figure 7–1), along with a few that follow a straight line, present several that include a junction (i.e., a V-shape), as in Figure 7–2 below. The junction shows the learner that changes can occasionally occur unexpectedly.

As part of this lesson, choose a visual symbol to represent the concept of an unwelcome surprise, such as a big red exclamation point. Refer to this visual symbol as the "big surprise," and display it near the junction, which shows the learner that the course of events changes when the big surprise appears (see Figure 7–2).

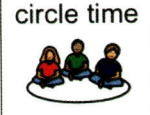  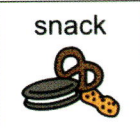 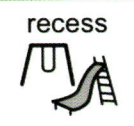 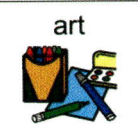 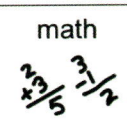

Figure 7–1. Example of a linear visual schedule. (From The Picture Communication Symbols ©1981–2007 by Mayer-Johnson LLC. All Rights Reserved Worldwide. Used with permission.

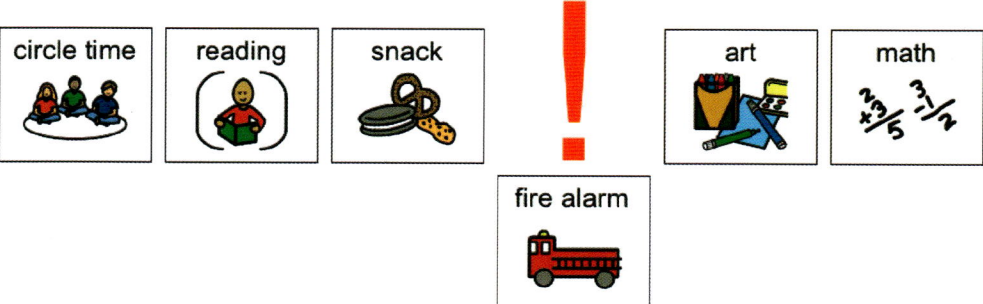

Figure 7–2. Example of a nonlinear display to account for surprise. (From The Picture Communication Symbols ©1981–2007 by Mayer-Johnson LLC. All Rights Reserved Worldwide. Used with permission.

Once the learner understands this lesson, you can apply the concept to real-life situations. When an unexpected event arises, show the learner a card with the big surprise symbol. You should also have another visual symbol available representing a preferred activity, such as a picture of an ice cream cone. So if the library is unexpectedly closed, you can point to the two visuals and say, "We can't go in the library today, but we'll go to the ice cream shop instead."

Two final points on controlling inappropriate behavior:

1. When a learner seems agitated and on the verge of acting out, you may be able to calm him by introducing activities that you know from prior experience he finds engaging or enjoyable (a tactic known as redirection). Moving from a task he finds challenging and difficult to a pleasant one (such as his favorite game) for a few minutes may avert a meltdown. In the long run, however, you should not let the fear of outbursts stop you from encouraging the learner to develop new skills (which, unfortunately, is a common occurrence). With proper use of a range of visual supports that clearly indicate a task's requirements and duration, you are greatly increasing the likelihood that individuals with ASD can sustain their attention and gradually learn increasingly complex skills.

2. Finally, it is important to recognize that the VIP cannot control all inappropriate behavior. Some outbursts result from causes other than the learner's inability to communicate (such as pain from an earache or anxiety associated with an activity), and in some cases the cause is impossible to detect. Even so, in our experience learners who use the VIP often show a sharp reduction in inappropriate behavior. Visual supports provide an expressive and receptive avenue allowing the child to focus better and enjoy activities and interactions with other people.

Expression of Pain and Discomfort

Chris exhibited frequent self-injurious, head banging behavior that resulted in a detached retina. His annual health screening revealed that he had been suffering from chronic ear infections. Regrettably his inability to express his extreme discomfort resulted in the loss of vision.

Individuals with ASD often do not report discomfort and pain and parents or instructors are first alerted to pain and discomfort through self-injurious behavior. It is not clear why some individuals with ASD do not reveal pain. In fact, it has been speculated that some persons on the autism spectrum have a high tolerance for pain—an observation that has not been substantiated. The inability to make pain and discomfort known may be due to ineffective monitoring of sensory input (i.e., he may not recognize he is in pain until it is intolerable and too severe to endure). Furthermore, if the individual has difficulty perceiving similarity between experiences, he may not use his knowledge of receiving help and comfort when he was in pain to seek similar help when he is in immediate distress. The frustration parents feel toward their children's communication difficulties is exacerbated and frightening when their child cannot communicate pain. His inability to relay a critical diagnostic feature of an illness or his inability to communicate pain until there is a catastrophic event is naturally a source of considerable anxiety for all persons involved in the care of the individual.

Appendix D contains a series of suggestions for the introduction of specialized visuals to help the individual with ASD learn to report on his pain or discomfort. This approach was developed in cooperation with the Monarch School for Children with Autism in Shaker Heights, Ohio. The focal point of this program is to systematically instruct the learner in recognizing sensation and reporting on his discomfort and pain through the use of a specialized set of visual representations of his body.

The Inclusive Classroom

The Individuals with Disabilities in Education Act (IDEA), as amended in 1997, requires that students with disabilities be educated "to the maximum extent appropriate" in the "least restrictive environment." For many learners with ASD, this means spending some portion of their school day in regular education classrooms often with an instructor to assist them, a practice once known as mainstreaming and now often called inclusion.

Inclusion has benefits and drawbacks for learners with ASD. A major advantage is improved social opportunities and development: By sharing a classroom with typically developing students and observing typical behavior, communication patterns, and routines, learners with autism are more apt to learn to interact with their peers. As a result, they are more likely to develop friendships and less likely to feel isolated and stigmatized. Equally important, in ideal circumstances inclusion sets the stage for a better overall education.

Inclusion's biggest drawback is that the language level in the classroom and some classroom activities may be beyond learners' ability to comprehend or inappropriate to their current learning needs. When this is the case, learners cannot process the teacher's instruction and end up missing much of the content, thereby squandering the educational opportunity. Or they spend the bulk of time in class working in a corner with an instructor, largely defeating the purpose of inclusion.

Although individuals with ASD will always face obstacles in an inclusive classroom, use of visuals before and during class can maximize their development. Each learner's educational experience will vary depending on his comprehension, communication, and behavioral skills, but in general the VIP can help make the classroom an environment conducive to learning.

Previewing

A way to improve the likelihood for successful classroom inclusion is advance work known as previewing, the practice of going over class material one-on-one before the teacher actually presents it to the class. Previewing allows instructors in school or parents at home to debut information using language and visual supports the learner comprehends, at a pace that suits the learner. It also removes some of the element of surprise from the learner's classroom experience. As a result, he can more easily follow the lesson when the teacher presents it in the classroom, increasing his comprehension (and also reducing the likelihood of inappropriate behavior).

Successful previewing requires teachers, instructors, and, if possible, parents to work together diligently. Ideally, they should meet regularly to discuss what topics students will be working on in coming weeks, identify good topics to preview, and review relevant lesson plans, vocabulary, concepts, and so forth. The learner's instructor then previews the lessons with him at school and parents preview the material at home. In class, the instructor provides relevant visual cues as the teacher covers the material. Whenever feasible, the instructor can include the learner with ASD in classroom activities when he or she knows the learner has previewed a particular object or concept.

The specifics of previewing vary by age and the learner's abilities. For younger students, it may be more practical to go over most or all activities in advance, as classrooms for younger learners often tend to repeat the same activities. For example, kindergartners commonly gather in a circle and talk about the weather in the morning. To prepare for this, the instructor can preview visuals for the sun, rain, clouds, a raincoat, an umbrella, and so on. When the teacher or other students mention these elements, the instructor can refer to the relevant visual. Similarly, an exercise such as "show and tell" can be previewed by having the learner with ASD practice his presentation at home or at school using scene cues to present a favored item (such as a pet or a toy) or experience (such as going to the beach or the zoo).

With older learners, a two-tiered approach may be necessary, as it is not usually possible to preview every lesson due to time constraints, a rapidly evolving curriculum, and the fact that some lessons may be too difficult for the learner even if previewed. Instead, the instructor and the teacher can identify lessons the learner is most likely to benefit from for previewing and also plan separate simultaneous instruction about the topic at the learner's instructional level at other times. If possible, lessons should be identified several days in advance, as the instructor or parent will need time to prepare and preview the lesson and the learner may require extended time to master the material.

The level of detail depends on the learner's comprehension skills. When previewing a science lesson on reptiles for a sixth grader, for example, the instructor should identify as many elements of the lesson as the learner is likely to comprehend and preview those in the days before the classroom lesson. If the learner has limited comprehension skills, the instructor can focus on providing visuals for two or three reptiles and a few relevant elements (such as habitat and some actions). More advanced learners may be able to handle dozens of element and scene cues.

Using Visuals Inside and Outside the Home

Parents should play an active role in the VIP, meeting with school officials regularly and helping preview upcoming class material. However, previewing is just one potential aspect of parents' participation. For the VIP to have maximum effect, visuals should be integrated into the child's entire life—at school, at home, and out in the world.

We do not mean to suggest that everything the child does must incorporate visuals. This is unrealistic—it is impossible to have a visual array prepared for every possible action or event, and, given the inherent demands of parenting a child with ASD, parents will not always have the time or energy to employ visuals for every occasion or activity.

Even so, many excellent opportunities exist for parents to use visual supports to promote language and comprehension growth. As described in Chapter 6, parents can help build a symbol-rich environment, associating common household objects with visual cues such as photographs, drawings, and text. These cues can be incorporated into daily routines, such as when the parent directs the child to get his coat, put away his toys, pour himself a glass of juice, brush his teeth, and so forth. The more visual symbols the learner encounters, the more likely he is to expand his vocabulary, recognize and use labels for objects, and apply this knowledge in novel contexts.

Whole scenes and scene cues can be used at home to prepare the child for experiences such as a trip to the library or mall or the arrival of a babysitter. Preparing a visual display in advance of a new experience, such as a visit to a new doctor's office or the child's first ferry ride, is especially helpful. It is also important to identify difficult situations, paying special attention to preparing the learner for experiences likely to upset him.

Similarly, visuals also can be used outside the home. For example, using a visual display during a trip to the zoo increases the chances that the learner will be able to identify zoo animals when he sees them in other situations (e.g., in a movie, video game, or book). During a long drive, parents can encourage the child to review his favorite whole scene displays or to match sights he sees through the car window to pictures from his whole scene or conversation displays. Such activities can make potentially difficult journeys into learning experiences.

We encounter a range of responses when we encourage parents to use visuals with their children. Although many parents are receptive, some parents say they do not need to use visuals because they can tell what their child wants from his actions. Parents with this mindset try to anticipate most of their child's needs. Often they organize the home to reduce the need for using symbols for communication, laying out frequently used items in easily accessible places.

Although it is true that parents are often adept at interpreting their children's behavior, the lack of a visual support system can be limiting, particularly if the learner needs to communicate anything out of his ordinary repertoire of requests or if he requires something outside of the immediate physical environment. Also, this position overlooks the fact that there is much more to communication than requesting. Ultimately, parents who decline to use visuals forfeit a prime opportunity for a child to improve his communication and comprehension skills and become more independent (he is unlikely to do so if his parents assume they always know what he wants). In the big picture, the VIP benefits learners with ASD if used in school or at home, but those who use the approach both at school and at home stand to make the greatest gains.

Intervention for Pre-Level I Learners

As discussed in Chapter 5, most individuals with ASD fall into three categories based on the Experiential Knowledge Profile, with Level I learners having the most difficulty performing routines and communicating. However, there is also a subset of the ASD population that lacks many of the basic skills of Level I learners. These individuals—whom we will refer to as Pre-Level I learners—do not understand the concept of cause and effect and cannot communicate with symbolic material even for the simplest requests. In this case, it is necessary for instructors and parents to interpret intent based on behavior. Following are some ways in which visuals can be used to help Pre-Level I learners improve communication skills.

Provide Frequent Opportunities for Learning Cause and Effect

Use of visuals can help Pre-Level I learners make the connection between simple actions and their consequences. For example, you can show learners computer screen displays in which pressing a key leads to an immediate visual response, such as a burst of color or the appearance of a cartoon character. Numerous mainstream toys are available that illustrate cause and effect, such as those that require the child to pull a string, push a button, wind a crank, or set a timer to prompt a sound, play a song, make a character pop up, and so forth. You also can use appliances and musical instruments to demonstrate cause and effect, such as by turning on a light switch or a fan or hitting a key on a piano, or purchase cause/effect toys designed especially for individuals with special learning needs. Bear in mind that Pre-Level I learners may be slow to grasp cause and effect, so it is important to demonstrate the concept as often as possible throughout the day. Two final points regarding cause and effect:

1. The instructor should select materials that match the learner's sensory interests. In other words, for the learner who is interested in auditory stimuli, music and environmental sounds should be the response when the learner activates a toy/switch.
2. Learners become bored or disinterested when materials are not varied. Even the most reinforcing toys can lose their learning impact if the toy no longer holds the interest of the learner.

Use Behavioral Interpretation to Lead into Teaching Basic Communication Skills

When working with Pre-Level I learners, you first need to become a skilled interpreter of the individual's behavior to understand his requests and protests. Once you recognize how he acts when he wants something, you can begin working on associating a gesture or movement to each request. For example, the learner may be able to learn to point to the sink when he is thirsty or stand by the cabinet containing preferred snacks to indicate his desire for food.

Introduce "Operant Menus" of Preferred Items

Pre-level I learners tend to have a paucity of material in which they show interest. As a result, it is difficult to introduce visual cues they can use to signal their desire for reinforcing items. To jump-

start this process, prepare an "operant menu"—a display of a collection of sensory materials or items the learner might be interested in. In selecting items, try to disregard what you personally believe to be interesting and introduce a variety of items that simply have sensorial appeal to the learner. Possibilities include toys that provide a range of musical and environmental sounds, objects with various textures, visually attractive items, and toys that move and vibrate. Once you present the menu, you can determine which items the learner prefers. Then you can introduce visual cues that stand for those items and begin the process of teaching the learner to request or use them as reinforcers.

Use Basic Matching Exercises

Exercises that use actual objects and highly iconic representations of these objects are an important step toward helping Pre-Level I learners move from communicating with gestures to using more abstract symbols. Items with eye-catching product logos can be useful here because learners often react to them. For example, many learners like to eat cereal for a snack and become excited when they see a cereal box, and some stand by the cabinet where the box is stored when they are hungry.

In such cases, start by placing the cereal box on a table close enough for the learner to reach and encourage him to grab it when he wants a snack. Once he can do this, place the box at increasing distances so he has to intentionally act on acquiring it. Next, replace the full box with an empty box, and show him that when he picks up the empty box, he still gets the snack. Once the learner understands the association between the full box and the empty box, you can introduce a 3D version (i.e., the front cover of the cereal box pasted onto a similarly sized box or piece of Styrofoam). Encourage the learner to bring the 3D version to you (or point to it) when he wants a snack, rewarding him when he does so. Such exercises set the stage for more advanced use of object elements and gestures, that is, eventually the child may learn to request items by using other types of symbolic representation.

Place Photos to Begin to Teach Labels

Creating a symbol-rich environment in which commonly used items have detachable photos on them may help Pre-Level I individuals learn the names of objects and begin to recognize them in different contexts. Please refer to Chapter 6 for suggestions on how to create a symbol-rich environment.

Intervention for Learners Who Read

Learners with ASD differ greatly in their overall reading skills. Among those who can read, their comprehension level varies widely, from reading aloud without comprehension to being able to comprehend written material better than spoken language. When learners demonstrate even minimal understanding that written words carry meaning, written language presents opportunities for improving comprehension (and, as a result, daily function) and promoting long-term language development. This section covers some strategies for taking advantage of these opportunities.

Improving Comprehension

Written language can be used to support spoken routine-based directives during daily activities. Although the nature of spoken language is transient—once a message is stated there is no physical imprint to refer to—a written version provides learners with a sustained referent that allows them to process information at their own pace. As a result, they are more likely to successfully act on the directive.

For example, some learners may not respond to the statement, "It's time to put on your coat, grab your backpack, and line up for the bus," because the spoken message passes too quickly for them to comprehend. In such cases, providing written instructions is likely to improve comprehension of the entire directive.

You can create a series of such written instructions for common routines and tasks. Bear in mind that when your goal is to use written language to support existing comprehension skills (not expand language skills), it is critical to use concepts, vocabulary, and syntax the learner understands. Your choices here should be based on the results of the VIP assessment (see Chapter 4). Using the findings of the reading skills assessment ensures that written information is composed of sight words or decodable text the learner is able to read.

You should also determine if it is advisable to restate written information aloud after the learner reads it. For some readers this may be a distraction but for others this additional spoken support may reinforce the message, increasing comprehension.

Promoting Long-Term Language Development

To improve language skills, we recommend writing short language development stories about familiar routines and topics of interest to the learner.[1] These stories establish a predictable context for the learner to improve and increase language skills (Gray, n.d.). Pictures that serve as visual supports should be incorporated into the stories whenever possible, as they may help the learner retrieve a well-known experience and apply his understanding of the procedures involved in executing the routine. For example, to teach the preposition "on," you might design a story centered on the routine of placing weather icons (e.g., sun, clouds, rain) on the calendar. The story can include a photograph of the learner placing an icon on the calendar with the caption: "John puts the sun *on* the calendar."

In general, you should use sentences that include words and concepts the learner already knows, plus language elements targeted for him to acquire. Initially, focus on one aspect of language development until the learner demonstrates proficiency with that particular skill. As the learner acquires each skill, create stories that continue to incorporate all newly acquired skills. This gives the learner

opportunities to practice the new skills, which helps him maintain them.

There are several factors to consider when deciding how to choose written words for these stories. The instructor should review the results of the reading skills assessment portion of the VIP to ascertain the learner's reading level and how he tends to acquire reading vocabulary. If the learner decodes well, you can choose words that can be easily sounded out to incorporate into the story. If he learned to read by associating whole words to objects or pictures, choose words from this existing sight word inventory to use within the story.

You should use words you know the learner already reads well and gradually add others relevant to the context of the story. If the learner reads aloud, it can be helpful to rehearse reading the story with him until he has demonstrated sufficient fluency in reading the text.

The level of syntax introduced in the stories should not exceed the level of syntactic understanding determined in the learner's VIP assessment. Instruction typically should begin with simple subject/verb/object sentences, such as "Sue eats her snack." As the learner acquires concepts such as descriptors (e.g., color, shape, and size), ordinal language (e.g., first, second), or temporal markers (e.g., before, after), add them into the basic subject/verb/object form. For example, the initial sentence of "Mary put the sun on the calendar" could be expanded to, "First, Mary put the big, yellow sun on the calendar."

---

[1] "Social stories," a concept developed by Carol Gray in which stories are used to help learners with ASD understand behavioral expectations, established a precedent for using stories as an instructional tool (Gray, n.d.).

Following are some suggestions for focusing on particular aspects of language development and comprehension:

Vocabulary

To expand the learner's noun vocabulary, write a story that includes vocabulary central to a certain topic. You may wish to begin with nouns because they are more concrete, most easily imaged, and provide multiple opportunities for associations. For example, you might write a story about a trip to the zoo that adds words like chimp, panther, and buffalo to familiar words like monkey, lion, and tiger. Similarly, verbs might expand from eat, sleep, and run to less common words like snack, rest, and exercise.

Concepts

Language development stories also lend themselves to building concept awareness. Routines that have sequences are ideal for teaching concepts of "first, next, last." For example, a story about snack time could read "*First*, Tom gets his snack from his cubby. *Next*, he sits at the table with his friends and eats his snack. *Last*, Tom throws his trash away in the pail."

Concepts such as "before and after" can be written into a story based on a well-known sequence or routine, for example, "Mary gets her backpack from her cubby *before* she gets on the bus. Mary gets on the bus *after* she gets her backpack."

Stories also can be used to expand vocabulary related to a specific concept. Start with a concept the learner understands, such as size. If he is familiar with small and big, work on increasing his understanding of more subtle gradations, such as tiny, medium, and huge.

Pragmatic Understanding

Reading is an excellent tool for increasing the learner's awareness of other people's perspectives. We find it helpful to construct two parallel versions of a well-rehearsed routine in the learner's life. For example, you might prepare a story about the learner's typical morning from both his point of view and his mother's. On the left-hand page, describe the mother's experience:

Mom Says
- "Wake up and come to the kitchen."
- "What do you want for breakfast?"
- "It's time to get dressed for school."

On the right-hand page, describe the learner's perspective on these same events:

My Morning
- John gets out of bed and walks to the kitchen.
- John wants pancakes with juice.
- John puts on his jeans, and T-shirt.

Another useful technique is to use a color-coded scheme to emphasize a particular aspect of the story, such as people, actions, or places. Include follow-up questions that correspond with the relevant color-coded information. Color-coding is especially helpful for teaching learners to understand "wh" words—what, who, where, when, why. For example, the *red* text in Table 7–1 emphasizes "what."

Table 7–1. Color Coding Suggestions

Bob wanted to see the Red Sox at Fenway Park.	Dad bought tickets to see the Red Sox at Fenway Park.
What did Bob want?	What did Dad do?

Color-coding that corresponds a "wh" word to its answer within the text allows you to bring the learner's attention immediately to the salient information. For example, you might prepare a story about a classroom activity, putting the "what" in *red*, the "where" in *green*, and the "who" in *blue*.

John gets his calendar and marker and sits on the rug.

Who gets his calendar and marker?

What does John get?

Where do John and the children sit?

If the learner has trouble answering the questions, he can use the colors to help guide him to the proper response (with the instructor's assistance if necessary). As the learner becomes proficient, you can begin fading use of colors and picture supports and start asking questions that require him to fill in a missing piece (i.e., the cloze procedure), such as: "John and the children sit _____." The ultimate goal is to fade all supports and have the learner successfully respond to an open-ended question such as "*Where does John sit?*"

Selecting Appropriate Assistive Technology

You face important but difficult technology decisions when building an intervention plan for a learner with autism: Would an augmentative and alternative communication (AAC) device help this individual express himself better?[2] If so, which device is likely to help him most? In this section, after a brief review of the history that led to the use of AAC devices by learners with autism, we offer a questionnaire (Appendix E) that can help you systematically address these complex issues.

Background

Current use of assistive communication devices[3] for learners with ASD stems from several trends that date back directly to the 1980s (with the groundwork laid in previous decades). Improvements in microprocessor technology in the 1980s made it feasible to develop and program computers with a range of communication applications. At the same time, a

---

[2]In terms of the VIP, AAC devices are primarily used for the Visual Expressive Mode (VEM). In some instances, these devices also enhance learners' ability to comprehend instructions (VIM) and organizational concepts (VOM).

[3]Other terms for assistive communication devices that use microprocessors include speech generating devices (SGDs) and electronic communication devices or aids.

nationwide movement aimed at ending warehousing of individuals with disabilities (deinstitutionalization) and providing opportunities for better education, social interaction, and employment took root. Legislation such as the Technology-Related Assistance for Individuals with Disabilities Act of 1988 (the "Tech Act") and the Americans with Disabilities Act of 1990 ensured that technology would play a key role in this movement.

Initially, AAC devices were used primarily to help people with motor control challenges, such as those with cerebral palsy and amyotrophic lateral sclerosis (Lou Gehrig's disease). In the 1990s, two developments led to the devices' use by learners with autism. First, PECS and other notebook-based augmentative communication methods demonstrated that visual supports were an effective tool for helping learners with ASD. Second, Facilitated Communication (FC), although controversial and ultimately proven invalid, generated interest in the idea that augmented communication strategies might benefit people with autism. (Chapter 1 includes further details on PECS and FC.)

Features of AAC Devices

In the last decade, AAC devices for people with ASD have proliferated. Hundreds of computers and standalone portable devices with specially designed screens and keyboards that allow the learner to view and manipulate images are now available. Although it is beyond the scope of this book to describe all the current devices, awareness of several distinguishing features can help you decide which device may be appropriate for a particular learner. Key issues that set one device apart from another include the following.

Dedicated Versus Computer-Based (General Purpose)

AAC devices may be dedicated (meaning they use a microprocessor designed exclusively as an assistive communication device) or computer-based (typically in the form of a laptop, tablet, or desktop, with a traditional operating system that runs communication-based software applications).

Traditional Keyboard Versus On-Screen Touch System

With a traditional keyboard, the learner types or presses buttons located beneath the screen. On-screen touch systems enable him to do so by touching a virtual keyboard displayed on a computer screen. Some devices include both options.

Static Screen Versus Dynamic Screen

Some devices can only display a single page of images at a time (e.g., photos, drawing, numbers, letters, etc.). Such static screen devices generally have a programmable surface that can accommodate both grid- and visual scene-based materials. Dynamic screen devices tend to be more feature rich, having a display screen that changes as a function of software demands and activation by a learner. A dynamic screen offers the learner the opportunity to organize symbolic content by categories and access information by branching to subpages. It is critical to know the device's capability in this regard, as it should match the levels of representation the learner understands.

Think of the dynamic screens as a computer screen and content changes as targets areas on the surface are selected.

The resulting images can be letters, graphics, animation, movies, and so forth.

A static screen on the other hand is more like an electronic bulletin board onto which materials can be adhered. The materials are external to the device and placed on top whereas a dynamic screen the images are stored internally.

Access Method

AAC devices may enable the learner to manipulate the visual symbols in a variety of ways, such as pointing and touching, pressing a button, or clicking a mouse.

Other Features

Some devices have been ruggedized to prevent breakage, and some have advanced audio capability to better support digital and/or synthetic speech output.

Making Key Decisions

Instructors should make decisions about AAC devices only after systemically evaluating the learner's needs (Shane & Bashir, 1980). Our questionnaire contains a decision matrix meant to help the instructor make informed choices.

Part 1: Deciding Whether to Use AAC

The first decision is whether or not a particular learner should use an AAC device. The choice needs be made on a case-by-case basis; many learners have no need for an assistive communication device, but others become more effec-tive communicators when they use one. (In our clinic, approximately 5% of learners use an electronic device for expressive communication purposes.[4]) That percentage rises dramatically when we consider the number of learners who use a computer for purposes of communication instruction.

Part 1 of the AAC Decision Questionnaire (Appendix E) elicits critical clinical information on the learner's current speech and communication skills, behavior, and previous experience with AAC devices. For each question, put a check mark in the Y (yes), N (no), U (uncertain), or N/A (not applicable) column.

In most cases, the questionnaire results do not provide a definitive answer. If there is a combination of yes and no responses and/or many uncertain responses, a trial may be useful in clarifying the appropriateness of using an AAC device. We recommend having the learner use the device for several weeks in multiple settings. At that point, the instructor can decide whether to continue use, based on whether he seems to be benefiting. If most or all answers are in the yes column, it is still a good idea to begin with an AAC trial, to confirm that initial indications were correct. If most or all answers are in the no column, AAC is probably not warranted.

Part 2: Choosing an Appropriate Device

If it is decided to use AAC for a particular learner, the next step is choosing which device to use. A critical aspect is knowing the levels of representation the learner can understand, which should be

---

[4]The prevalence of assistive communication device users is significantly higher when training for communication competence is included.

determine during the initial assessment of the learner's visual representation skills. Part 2 of the questionnaire (Appendix E) provides examples of specific device types that may be a good match for learners based on this assessment.

For example, a learner who reads might benefit from a device that allows for alphabet and word usage, whereas a learner who cannot read will at that point likely use a device that offers symbols rather than text as its graphic content.

The choice of a device should also take into account some practical issues. For example, does the learner need adult supervision when using the device, or can he use it by himself? Can the learner independently carry the device with him?

What uses besides communication might the learner use the device for (such as music and games)? The final section of the questionnaire helps you evaluate these issues.

References

Gray, C. (n.d.). *Social stories.* Kentwood, MI: The Gray Center for Social Learning and Understanding.

Shane H. C., & Bashir, A. S. (1980). Election criteria for determining candidates for an augmentative communication system. *Journal of Speech and Hearing Disorders, 45,* 408–414.

Monarch Natural Language Assessment

The Monarch Natural Language Assessment is used when a student does not have the executive skills necessary to participate in a standardized assessment, even though his primary mode of communication is spoken language. The Assessment is a checklist of verbal skills that is filled out at the student's first staffing, so parents and staff can work together to document the student's spoken language behaviors across different environments.

_____

Name   Age   Date

Reactional Language

- ☐ is able/unable to respond appropriately to well-rehearsed, frequently presented words and phrases (e.g., his name, and directives such as "come here," and "no").
- ☐ reliably/unreliably ceases activity when his name is called, when he sees a visual, or hears the word "stop."
- ☐ is able/unable to understand specific routine phrases such as "go get your shoes by identifying the noun "shoes" and anticipating the routine attached to it.

Indication

- ☐ is able/unable to use a pointing gesture to indicate recognition of an object/picture (contact point).
- ☐ is able/unable to use a pointing gesture to refer to an object/visual for requesting or commenting (contact point).
- ☐ is able/unable to use a distal point for capturing the attention of another person.
- ☐ can/cannot respond appropriately to yes/no questions involving a choice of preferred/nonpreferred items.

☐ is able/unable to indicate that he needs assistance through a verbal response, a gesture, or through the use of visual symbols.

☐ is able/unable to indicate that he is experiencing pain or discomfort through a verbal response, a gesture, or through the use of a graphic.

☐ is able/unable to request people and/or items that are not in his immediate environment.

Labeling

☐ is able/unable to label nouns/actions/functions.

☐ is able/unable to sort nouns by category and function.

☐ is able/unable to direct his attention to the outdoor environment to comment on and label the weather.

☐ is able/unable to comment on his health (e.g., reporting an earache, stomachache, or headache).

☐ is able/unable to comment on his own emotional state (e.g., "I am angry at John").

☐ is able/unable to refer to himself by his own name.

☐ is able/unable to use appropriate pronouns to refer to himself and others.

☐ is able/unable to demonstrate understanding and use of the plural form.

☐ is able/unable to demonstrate understanding and use of indication/control language, such as touch, point to, show me, stop, and wait.

Activation/Cessation

☐ is able/unable to demonstrate understanding and use of safety related commands, such as stop, don't, and quiet hands.

☐ is able/unable to respond to and use vocabulary related to seeking, such as find, look for, and "where is?"

☐ is able/unable to understand and use vocabulary related to requesting, such as give me, please, and may I.

☐ is able/unable to understand and use vocabulary related to transfer actions, such as give, put, and get.

☐ is able/unable to understand and use vocabulary related to body actions, such as run, jump, sit, stand up, and leave.

☐ is able/unable to demonstrate understanding and use of ADL vocabulary, such as brush, comb, wash, wipe, eat, chew, swallow, and drink.

Attribution

☐ is able/unable to recognize and describe by descriptors, such as color, size, shape, texture, and weight.

☐ is able/unable to use locative prepositions, such as on, under, in, out, next to behind, in front of.

☐ is able/unable to demonstrate understanding and use of vocabulary related to directions, such as first, second, middle, last; and distance, such as near and far.

☐ is able/unable to describe by comparison, such as good, better, best, biggest, smaller.

☐ is able/unable to demonstrate understanding of time and sequence, such as days of the week, months of the year, seasons of the year; and concepts, such as yesterday, today and tomorrow, five more minutes, and morning, afternoon, and evening.

☐ is able/unable to demonstrate knowledge of spatial/directional skills, such as left, right, straight, near, and turn.

Quantitative

☐ is able/ unable to use vocabulary related to understanding quantity, such as, how much, more, and less.

Interpretation

☐ is able/unable to demonstrate understanding and use of "wh" questions of who, where, what, when, and how.

☐ is able/unable to understand and use the reverse interrogative question form.

☐ is able/unable to apply backward inferencing to a sequence of events in order to explain the outcome of the sequence.

☐ is able/unable to apply forward inferencing to a series of events in order to predict the outcome.

Following Directions

☐ is able/unable to follow one/two/ multistep directions.

☐ is able/unable to understand and apply knowledge of elements, such as color, size, shape, texture, weight.

☐ is able/unable to understand temporal markers, such as before, after, and while.

☐ demonstrates a recency/latency effect in response to directions; typically responds to the last/first item that was presented in a sequence.

Pragmatics

☐ is able/unable to pick up on social clues and initiate the appropriate use of greetings and partings.

☐ is able/unable to initiate a conversation with his peers and/or adults.

☐ is able to maintain topic for _____ conversational turns.

☐ is able/unable to comment on the emotional state of others, such as "John looks unhappy."

☐ is able/unable to appropriately switch topics.

☐ consistently/inconsistently requests clarification when he is unsure of the intended meaning of his conversational partner.

Intelligibility

(When appropriate)

APPENDIX B

Informal Language Milestones

Question Form	Age (Years-Months)	Concept	Structured Response
1. Yes/No	2-0		
2. What + be	2-0	Identity	Noun
3. What + do	2-6	Action	Verb
4. Where (place)	2-6	Space	Adverb, prepositional phrase
5. Where (direction)	2-6	Location	Noun, prepositional phrase
6. Who	2-6	Person	Noun, pronoun
7. Whose	2-6	Possession	Possessive pronoun or markers
8. Why	3-0	Cause/effect	Because phrases
9. How	3-6	Manner-method	Adverb
many-few	3-0	Number	
much-little	3-6	Quantity	
long-short	4-0	Duration	
far-near	4-6	Distance	
often-soon	5-0	Time	
long-short	5-6	Linear	
big-small	5-6	Size	
10. When	5-6	Time	Adverb, tense, prepositional phrase
11. Which	5-6	Selection	This/that, multiple choice

Source: Age of acquisition of yes-no interrogatives and wh-questions by typical language learners from Chapman (1981).

131

Experiential Knowledge Profile (EKP)

Kitchen Routines

	Beverage Routine	Learner-Acquired				Adult-Directed			
		Mastered	In Progress	Prompted		Mastered	In Progress	Prompted	N/A
A-1	**Move** to the refrigerator								
B-1	**Open** the refrigerator door								
C-1	**Get** the container								
D-1	**Close** the refrigerator door								
B-2	**Open** the cupboard door								
C-2	**Get** the glass/cup								
D-2	**Close** the cupboard door								
E-1	**Put** the glass on the table								
B-3	**Open** the container								
F-1	**Transfer** the beverage into the glass								

	Snack Routine	Learner-Acquired				Adult-Directed			
		Mastered	In Progress	Prompted		Mastered	In Progress	Prompted	N/A
B-4	**Open** *the cupboard*								
C-3	**Get** *the snack bag out of the cupboard*								
D-3	**Close** *the cupboard door*								
B-5	**Open** *the bag*								
G-1	**Consume** *the snack*								
H-1	**Insert** *the bag into the trash (wastebasket)*								

	Handwashing Routine	Learner-Acquired				Adult-Directed			
		Mastered	In Progress	Prompted		Mastered	In Progress	Prompted	N/A
A-2	**Move** *to the sink*								
K-1	**Activate** *the faucet*								
C-4	**Get** *the soap*								
L-1	**Position** *hands under the water*								
M-1	**Replace** *the soap*								
L-2	**Position** *hands under the water*								
N-1	**Deactivate** *the faucet*								
C-5	**Get** *the towel*								
O-1	**Wipe** *hands*								
M-2	**Replace** *the towel*								

	Sitting at Kitchen Table Routine	Learner-Acquired				Adult-Directed			
		Mastered	In Progress	Prompted		Mastered	In Progress	Prompted	N/A
E-2	**Put** *the tableware on the table*								
L-3	**Position** *oneself in the chair*								
L-4	**Position** *the chair at the table*								
L-5	**Position** *the fork and spoon appropriately*								
O-2	**Wipe** *with the napkin*								
C-6	**Get** *the dishes from the table*								
E-3	**Put** *the dishes in the sink*								

Bathroom Routines

	Hand Washing Routine	Learner-Acquired				Adult-Directed			
		Mastered	In Progress	Prompted		Mastered	In Progress	Prompted	N/A
A-3	**Move** *to the sink*								
K-2	**Activate** *the faucet*								
C-7	**Get** *the soap*								
E-4	**Put** *hands under the water*								
M-3	**Replace** *the soap*								
L-6	**Position** *hands under the water*								
N-2	**Deactivate** *the faucet*								
C-8	**Get** *the towel*								
O-3	**Wipe** *hands*								
M-4	**Replace** *the towel*								

	Toothbrushing Routine	Learner-Acquired				Adult-Directed			
		Mastered	In Progress	Prompted		Mastered	In Progress	Prompted	N/A
A-4	**Move** *to the sink*								
C-9	**Get** *the toothbrush*								
C-10	**Get** *the toothpaste*								
B-6	**Open** *the toothpaste*								
F-2	**Transfer** *the toothpaste on the toothbrush*								
D-4	**Close** *the toothpaste*								
M-5	**Replace** *the toothpaste*								
P-1	**Personal Care** *(mouth)*								
P-2	**Personal Care** *(mouth)*								
L-7	**Position** *the toothbrush under the water*								
M-6	**Replace** *the toothbrush*								

	Toileting Routine	Learner-Acquired				Adult-Directed			
		Mastered	In Progress	Prompted		Mastered	In Progress	Prompted	N/A
A-5	**Move** *to the toilet*								
Q-1	**Undress** *self*								
L-8	**Position** *self on the toilet*								
O-4	**Wipe** *with toilet paper*								
H-2	**Insert** *toilet paper into the toilet*								
L-9	**Position** *self off the toilet*								
R-1	**Dress** *self*								
K-3	**Activate** *toilet flushing*								
	Wash Hands *(refer to hand-washing routine)*								

	Bathtub Routine	Learner-Acquired				Adult-Directed			
		Mastered	In Progress	Prompted		Mastered	In Progress	Prompted	N/A
D-5	**Close** *the water drain*								
K-4	**Activate** *the faucet*								
F-3	**Transfer** *bubble bath into the bath water*								
Q-2	**Undress** *self*								
A-6	**Move** *into the tub*								
N-3	**Deactivate** *the faucet*								
P-3	**Use** *washcloth and soap*								
S-1	**Play** *with bathtub toys*								
A-7	**Move** *self out of the tub*								
O-5	**Wipe** *with the towel*								
R-2	**Dress** *self*								
B-7	**Open** *the water drain*								

Bedroom Routines

	Putting Away Toys Routine	Learner-Acquired				Adult-Directed			
		Mastered	In Progress	Prompted		Mastered	In Progress	Prompted	N/A
B-8	**Open** *the toy chest/closet/ cabinet door*								
C-11	**Get** *the toys*								
M-7	**Replace** *the toys*								
D-6	**Close** *the toy chest/closet/ cabinet door*								

	Dressing for the Day Routine	Learner-Acquired				Adult-Directed			
		Mastered	In Progress	Prompted		Mastered	In Progress	Prompted	N/A
B-9	**Open** *the drawers/closet door*								
C-12	**Get** *clothing*								
D-7	**Close** *the closet/cabinet door*								
R-3	**Dress** *clothing*								
R-4	**Dress** *footwear*								

	Undressing Routine	Learner-Acquired				Adult-Directed			
		Mastered	In Progress	Prompted		Mastered	In Progress	Prompted	N/A
Q-3	Undress *footwear*								
Q-4	Undress *clothing*								
B-10	Open *the hamper*								
E-5	Put *clothing into the hamper*								
D-8	Close *the hamper*								

	Dressing for Bed Routine	Learner-Acquired				Adult-Directed			
		Mastered	In Progress	Prompted		Mastered	In Progress	Prompted	N/A
B-11	Open *the drawers/closet door*								
C-13	Get *pajamas/ nightgown*								
R-5	Dress *night clothes*								
D-9	Close *the closet/cabinet door*								

Living Room Routines

	Using a TV Routine	Learner-Acquired				Adult-Directed			
		Mastered	In Progress	Prompted		Mastered	In Progress	Prompted	N/A
K-5	**Activate** *power for the TV*								
I-1	**Determine** *the channel*								
I-2	**Determine** *volume*								
M-8	**Deactivate** *the TV*								

	Using a Video/ DVD Routine	Learner-Acquired				Adult-Directed			
		Mastered	In Progress	Prompted		Mastered	In Progress	Prompted	N/A
K-6	**Activate** *power for the video/ DVD player*								
H-3	**Insert** *video/ DVD into the player*								
K-7	**Activate** *play for the video/ DVD player*								
K-8	**Activate** *video/ DVD controls*								
C-14	**Get** *video/DVD from the player*								

	Using a Computer Routine	Learner-Acquired				Adult-Directed			
		Mastered	In Progress	Prompted		Mastered	In Progress	Prompted	N/A
K-9	**Activate** *power for the computer*								
K-10	**Activate** *the mouse pointer*								
K-11	**Activate** *the computer activity*								

Classroom Routines

	Snacking Routine: Drinking from a juice box	Learner-Acquired				Adult-Directed			
		Mastered	In Progress	Prompted		Mastered	In Progress	Prompted	N/A
C-15	**Get** *the beverage box from the cubby*								
B-12	**Open** *the box*								
H-4	**Insert** *the straw into the container*								
G-2	**Consume** *the beverage*								
H-5	**Insert** *the container into the trash*								

	Snacking Routine: Eating from a snack bag	Learner-Acquired				Adult-Directed			
		Mastered	In Progress	Prompted		Mastered	In Progress	Prompted	N/A
C-16	**Get** *the snack bag from the cubby*								
B-13	**Open** *the bag*								
L-10	**Position** *oneself in the chair*								
L-11	**Position** *the chair at the table*								
G-3	**Consume** *the snack*								
H-6	**Insert** *the bag in the trash*								

	Tabletop Activity Routine	Learner-Acquired				Adult-Directed			
		Mastered	In Progress	Prompted		Mastered	In Progress	Prompted	N/A
L-12	**Position** *oneself in the chair*								
L-13	**Position** *the chair at the table*								
T-1	**Attend** *to the teacher*								
U-1	**Work** *on the task*								
F-4	**Transfer** *the work to the teacher*								

	Entering and Greeting: School Routine	Learner-Acquired				Adult-Directed			
		Mastered	In Progress	Prompted		Mastered	In Progress	Prompted	N/A
A-8	**Move** *down the bus stairs*								
V-1	**Greet** *staff members*								
A-9	**Move** *toward the school*								
B-14	**Open** *the school building door*								
A-10	**Move** *down the hallway*								
V-2	**Greet** *teachers and other students*								
Q-5	**Undress** *coat/ sweater/hoody*								
E-6	**Put** *backpack in the cubby*								
B-15	**Open** *the classroom door*								
A-11	**Move** *into the classroom*								

		Learner-Acquired				Adult-Directed			
	Exiting and Parting: School Routine	Mastered	In Progress	Prompted		Mastered	In Progress	Prompted	N/A
W-1	**Part** *from staff and students*								
A-12	**Move** *out of the classroom*								
C-17	**Get Dressed** *coat/sweater/ hoody out of the cubby*								
C-18	**Get** *backpack out of the cubby*								
A-13	**Move** *out of the classroom*								
A-14	**Move** *down the hallway*								
B-16	**Open** *the school building door*								
A-15	**Move** *to the bus*								
A-16	**Move** *up the bus stairs*								

Function Key

	Kitchen	Bathroom	Bedroom	Living Room	Classroom
Move	A-1, A-2	A-3, A-4, A-5, A-6, A-7			A-8, A-9, A-10, A-11, A-12, A-13, A-14, A-15, A-16
Put	E-1, E-2, E-3	E-4	E-5		E-6
Transfer	F-1	F-2, F-3			F-4
Consume	G-1				G-2, G-3
Insert	H-1	H-2		H-3	H-4, H-5, H-6
Determine				I-1, I-2	
Position	L-1, L-2, L-3, L-4, L-5	L-6, L-7, L-8, L-9			L-10, L-11, L-12, L-13
Wipe	O-1, O-2,	O-3, O-4, O-5			
Personal Care		P-1, P-2, P-3			
Undress		Q-1, Q-2	Q-3, Q-4		Q-5
Dress		R-1, R-2	R-3, R-4, R-5		
Play		S-1			
Attend					T-1
Work					U-1
Greet					V-1, V-2
Part					W-1

Initiation-Completion Skill Key

	Kitchen	Bathroom	Bedroom	Living Room	Classroom
Open	B-1, B-2, B-3, B-4, B-5	B-6, B-7	B-8, B-9, B-10, B-11		B-12, B-13, B-14, B-15, B-16
Close	D-1, D-2, D-3	D-4, D-5	D-6, D-7, D-8, D-9		
Get	C-1, C-2, C-3, C-4, C-5, C-6	C-7, C-8, C-9, C-10	C-11, C-12, C-13	C-14	C-15, C-16 C-17, C-18
Replace	M-1, M-2	M-3, M-4, M-5, M-6	M-7	M-8	
Activate	K-1	K-2, K-3, K-4		K-5, K-6, K-7, K-8, K-9, K-10, K-11	
Deactivate	N-1	N-2, N-3			

Summary

Functions

Number of Learner-Acquired Functions: /	Number of Adult-Directed Functions: /
Learner acquired functions, which are circled in *red*, were learned independently	Adult directed functions, which are circled in *blue*, were learned by explicit adult direction

Assist for Learner-Acquired Functions

Assist for Learner-Acquired Functions
These assists are used to retrieve or prompt an acquired function.
spoken:
gestural:
graphic:
written:

Assist for Adult-Directed Functions

Assist for Adult-Directed Functions
These assists are used to instruct while the Learner is acquiring the function
spoken:
gestural:
graphic:
written:
physical:

Completed Routines

Routines are considered completed if the learner performs a minimum of three steps ending with the last step in the routine.

Kitchen

	Complete
Beverage	
Snack	
Hand Washing	
Sitting at Kitchen Table	

Bathroom

	Complete
Washing Hands	
Toothbrushing	
Toileting	
Bathtub	

Bedroom

	Complete
Putting Away Toys	
Dressing for the Day	
Undressing	
Dressing for Bed	

Living Room

	Complete
Using a TV	
Using a VCR	
Using a Computer	

Classroom

	Complete
Snacking: drinking from a juice box	
Snacking: eating from a snack bag	

Juncture Expansion Vocabulary

Juncture Word	Expansion Words
move	climb down climb into climb out climb up exit get down get in get out go down go into go go in go to go out go up leave move walk walk in walk to walk out
open	lift pull push push up rip/tear slide turn, pull twist/turn/unscrew
get	grab pick up remove take out
close	pull up push push down shut slide tie twist/turn/screw on Velcro

continues

151

continued

Juncture Word	Expansion Words
put	hang up put in put on put under
transfer	bring give pour in scoop in serve squeeze on
consume	drink eat
insert	push put in throw away throw in
determine	change (as in station) change (as in volume) measure
mix	combine stir swirl
activate	click (mouse) contact (touchscreen) double-click (mouse) fast forward (VCR) flush move (mouse) pause (button) play pull up push down push in push out rewind stop touch (screen) turn turn on
position	hold pick up push in

Juncture Word	Expansion Words
position *(continued)*	put under sit in sit on stand up
replace	insert put back put down put in
deactivate	pull up push down push in push out turn
wipe	clean dry
personal care	bathe brush clean comb rinse shave shower
undress	pull down pull down pull off pull up take off unbutton undo Velcro unhook unsnap untie unzip
dress	button hook pull pull down pull on pull up put on snap zip

continues

continued

Juncture Word	Expansion Words
play	bounce build catch color draw jump make push scoop slide squeeze swing throw
attend	(you) do this listen look quiet hands quiet voice raise hand turn taking
work	cut draw imitate/copy match point read write/copy
greet	high five hug kiss say "Hi"
part	high five hug kiss say "Bye"

Noun Vocabulary

Category	Vocabulary
Bathroom items	bathtub bathtub plug bathtub toys brush bubble bath bubbles cap comb cup faucet mirror sink soap soap dish toilet toilet paper toothbrush toothbrush holder toothpaste towel washcloth
Bedroom items	bed bedspread blanket closet comforter drawers dresser hamper pillow quilt sheet toy toy chest
Clothing	backpack belt boots bra buttons coat dress gloves hat hoody hooks

continues

continued

Category	Vocabulary
Clothing *(continued)*	jacket mittens nightgown pajama bottoms pajama tops pants robe scarf shirt shoelaces shoes skirt slippers snaps snowpants socks sweater underpants undershirt velcro zipper
Food	bread butter cake carrot sticks celery sticks cheese cheese puffs chips cookies corn chips crackers gelatin ice cream jelly juice milk pasta pretzels pudding sandwich snack snack bag soda soup water yogurt

Category	Vocabulary
Kitchenware	bottle opener bowl cabinet can opener chair clock container counter cup cupboard dish soap dishcloth dishes dishtowel dishwasher drawers floor fork garbage garbage disposal glass knife napkins pans paper towels placemat plates pots refrigerator sink sponge spoon stove straw table tablecloth toaster wastebasket
Living Room items	CD channel button computer controls DVD lamps mouse

continues

continued

Category	Vocabulary
Living Room items *(continued)*	on/off (power) button program remote station stereo TV videotape VCR volume button
People items	brother bus driver Dad friend her him me Mom sister teacher you
School items	backpack book building bus chair classroom crayon cubby desk door eraser exit hallway marker paper pen pencil ruler school scissors stairs table whiteboard

Monarch Individualized Pain, Illness, and Discomfort Awareness Program[1]

Materials

- photograph of learner in bathing suit (front and back view)
- Band-Aids
- cold pack (e.g., chilled can of soda)
- warm compress
- nontoxic markers
- book of scene cues that depict an actor expressing different kinds of pain/illness/discomfort:
    - headache
    - earache
    - toothache
    - sore throat
    - chest pain
    - stomach pain
    - back pain
    - arm pain
    - hand/finger pain (infected cuticles)
    - leg pain
    - foot pain
    - toe pain (ingrown toe nails)

Body Awareness *(Instruction with visuals and spoken language[2] when appropriate)*

- Learner identifies his or her personal body photograph (front and back view)
- Learner identifies corresponding picture of body part when touched on his or her body
- Learner identifies corresponding body part on his or her body when presented with a picture of the body part

Identification of Visible Marks on Body

- Instructor draws marks on learner's arms, hand and/or legs with a washable nontoxic marker

---

[1]The Monarch pain awareness program was created in concert with the faculty from the Monarch School for Children with Autism in Shaker Heights, Ohio.

[2]Instructors should assess the learner's ability to use appropriate language to express pain. Language that the learner may already have associated with pain or discomfort such as "ouchy, boo-boo, hurt" should be mapped onto the instruction and encouraged.

- Instructor has learner identify the mark on his or her body
- Instructor demonstrates for the learner where the corresponding mark occurs on learner's personal body photograph
- Instructor has learner identify where the corresponding mark occurs on learner's personal body photograph

Identification of Sensation

- Instructor places either a "hand warmer," cold can of soda/water, or pressure on the same areas that were marked with the nontoxic washable markers
- Instructor demonstrates for the learner where the corresponding area occurs on learner's personal body photograph
- Instructor has learner identify where the corresponding area occurs on learner's personal body photograph

- Instructor places Band-Aid on the designated area on the learner's personal body photograph
- Learner places Band-Aid on the designated area on his or her personal body photograph
- Instructor places Band-Aid on the designated area on the learner

Visible Pain Graphics

- Instructor shows learner pictures of cuts, bruises, rashes, splinters, infected teeth, on a photograph of a neutral, unidentified person
- Instructor places a Band-Aid on the corresponding body part on the photograph of a neutral, unidentified person
- Learner places the Band-Aid on the corresponding body part on the photograph of a neutral, unidentified person

Key Factors in Selecting an Electronic Communication Device

Section 1: Deciding Whether to Use AAC

Speech Production	Yes (**Y**): AAC Indicated	No (**N**): AAC not indicated	Uncertain (**U**): Examine clinically and return to the question	N/A
1. Is this individual's speech ineffective in most speaking situations?				
2. Does this individual produce a limited amount of speech?				
3. Is this individual's speech mostly unintelligible?				
4. Does this individual self-limit speech production?				
5. Has it been observed since the introduction of visual supports that this individual tends to produce more speech?				
6. Has it been observed since the introduction of visual supports that this individual is attempting to speak?				
7. Does this individual speak or attempt to speak while pointing to photos, graphic symbols, or words?				
Communication				
Intent				
1. Does this individual seem frustrated because he or she is unable to get his/her needs met?				
2. Is this individual aware that intentionally pointing to, handing over, or indicating some representation is the means to acquire an item?				
3. Does this individual bring you to the location of a desired item or activity?				

Behavior Do you suspect that aggressive or self-injurious behaviors, if they occur, are related to difficulty with communicating related to:	**Y:** AAC Indicated	**N:** AAC not indicated	**U:** Carefully monitor behavior	**N/A**
inability to request activities				
desire to escape				
ineffectiveness at asking that an activity continue or stop				
need for attention				
sensory over/understimulation				

Recognition/Representation Level Does this individual recognize that an object can be represented by (Please indicate all that apply):	**Y:** Introduce AAC at least at this level of representation	**N:** AAC not indicated	**U:** Continue sampling and revisit the question	**N/A**
miniature objects				
3D photos				
Photographs				
colored drawings				
line drawings				
text/whole words				
text/alpha-numeric				
scene-based material				
actions through animation				
actions through live movies				

Prior AAC Experience

Low-Tech Experience

	Y: Consider trial with hi-tech device	N: Continue training with lo-tech approach	U: Continue sampling and revisit the question	N/A
1. Has this individual successfully used a graphic symbol approach, e.g., Picture Exchange Communication System (PECS) to request, label, or comment?				
2. Has this individual successfully used manual signs or gestures to request, label, or comment?				

Hi-Tech Experience

	Y: Continue with device or consider device with more advanced options	N: Continue training	U: Continue sampling and revisit the question	N/A
1. Has this individual had successful prior experience using a hi-tech communication device?				
2. Has this individual been more willing to communicate and become a more effective communicator with a hi-tech device?				

Question	Y	N	U	N/A
3. Was this individual's previous experience with a communication device unsuccessful because the speech output served more as a toy than a tool?	**Y:** Introduce training to help make that distinction	**N:** Continue with device or consider device with more advanced options	**U:** Continue sampling and revisit the question	**N/A**
4. Was this individual's previous experience with a communication device considered unsuccessful because the individual's communication was equally effective with and without the device?	**Y:** Consider device with more advanced options. If no improvement, continue with lo-tech device	**N:** Continue with device or consider device with more advanced options	**U:** Continue sampling and revisit the question	**N/A**
Communicative Intent Was this individual's previous experience with a communication device unsuccessful because the individual did not seem to recognize that the communication device (with speech output) was meant to serve as an expressive communication tool?	**Y:** Communication Device not indicated	**N:** Communication Device may be indicated	**U:** Continue sampling and revisit the question	**N/A**

Section 2: Choosing an Appropriate Device

Level of Representation Factors

Refer to the level of representation identified earlier to determine which device is a good match for this individual.

Level of Representation	Potential Device Type
miniature objects	
3D photos	• Static Screen Device
photographs	• Static Screen Device • Dynamic Screen Device • Static Screen Simulation • Dynamic Screen Simulation
colored drawings	• Static Screen Device • Dynamic Screen Device • Static Screen Simulation • Dynamic Screen Simulation
line drawings	• Static Screen Device • Dynamic Screen Device • Static Screen Simulation • Dynamic Screen Simulation
text/whole words	• Static Screen Device • Dynamic Screen Device • Static Screen Simulation • Dynamic Screen Simulation
text-alpha numeric	• Keyboard • Static Screen Device • Dynamic Screen Device • Static Screen Simulation • Dynamic Screen Simulation • Symbol/Word Arrangement • Text Box Arrangement
scene-based material	• Static Screen Display • Dynamic Screen Display • Static Screen Simulation • Dynamic Screen Simulation
actions through animation	• Dynamic Screen Device • Dynamic Screen Simulation
actions through live movie	• Dynamic Screen Device • Dynamic Screen Simulation

Electronic Device Factors

SUITABILITY

Behavior Does this individual have behavioral outbursts that:	Y: Introduce AAC with: • supervision and/or • ruggedization and/or • graduated training Goal is full device use	N: Introduce AAC. No need for ruggedization and/or supervision	U: Introduce and supervise to determine Y/N	N/A
could destroy the device				
necessitate a rugged device				
necessitate use of a device under adult supervision.				
	Y: AAC indicated	N: AAC not indicated	U: Examine clinically and revisit the question	N/A
Interest				
1. Does this individual look attentively at AAC devices used by other individuals?				
2. Has this individual spontaneously used another individual's AAC device for entertainment (e.g., including self-stimulating)?				
3. Has this individual spontaneously used another individual's AAC device to communicate?				

PORTABILITY	Y: Select AAC Device that is portable	N: Lo-Tech solution or engineer the environment	U: Gather further information and revisit the question	N/A
Could this individual independently transport a communication device?				
Is this individual aware of the need to carry the communication device with him/her?				

USE				
Interest	Y: Computer-based AAC device indicated	N: Dedicated or static AAC device indicated	U: Gather further information and revisit the question	N/A
1. In addition to using an AAC device for expressive communication, would this individual also use the device for other digital activities or experiences:				
listening to music				
watching videos/music videos				
playing games				
educational activities				
Web browsing				
E-mail				
2. Can this individual be engaged in a computer activity at home or in school for more than 3–5 minutes?				

	Y: Computer-based AAC device indicated	N: Dedicated or static AAC device indicated	U: Gather further information and revisit the question	N/A
3. Does this individual use the computer for entertainment?				
4. Does this individual enjoy using computer software that speaks the labels of objects when selected?				
5. Does this individual follow spoken directions given through the computer?				
6. Would consolidation of several low-tech or hi-tech options into one device be easier for this individual?				
Availability	Y: Computer-based or dedicated AAC device indicated	N: Computer-based AAC device indicated	U: Gather further information and revisit the question	N/A
7. Would a computer be available to this individual throughout the day to meet the necessities of these digital experiences?				

Index